HARVARD H
AND
ITS VOLUNTEERS

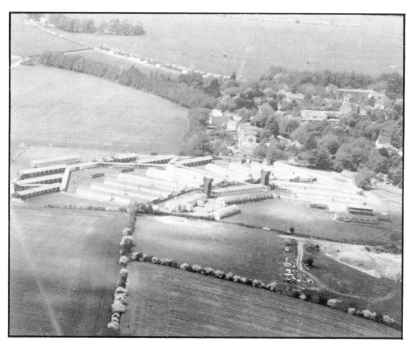

Aerial view of the Common Cold Research Unit (Harvard Hospital), at Salisbury, Wiltshire. (Photograph courtesy Aero Films and Aero Pictorial Ltd.)

HARVARD HOSPITAL AND ITS VOLUNTEERS

The Story Of
The Common Cold Research Unit

Keith R. Thompson

DANNY HOWELL BOOKS
MCMXC

Harvard Hospital And Its Volunteers
The Story of The Common Cold Research Unit

© Keith R. Thompson 1991

first published January 1991
by Danny Howell Books
57 The Dene, Warminster, Wiltshire, BA12 9ER

Design and Layout Conceived
by
Danny Howell

Typesetting, Photo-screening and Printing
by
Wessex Press Design & Print Limited
Graphic House, 55–57 Woodcock Industrial Estate,
Warminster, Wiltshire, BA12 9DY

Price: £8.50

ISBN 1 872818 04 8

Contents

Acknowledgements   7

Preface by Dr D. A. J. Tyrrell,
   C.B.E., M.D., D.S.E., F.R.C.P., F.R.C.Path., F.R.S. . .   9

Foreword by Dr A. T. Roden,
   Medical Superintendent at Harvard 1951–1956 . . .   11

Introduction   15

Joining The Unit   19

Preparation For The First Trial   21

Recruiting Of Volunteers   27

From Small Beginnings   33

Harvard's Directors   41

The Unit's Ten Medical Superintendents   43

Matrons Of Harvard   47

Kitchen And Catering   51

Volunteers, Why They Came And Their Comments . .   59

Cures And Curios   77

From The Scrapbook   85

The Ebble Valley Study   91

Seal Island Colds   95

Reflections 119

Appendix One — Buildings And Their Upkeep 125

Appendix Two — Both Volunteers And Staff 137

Appendix Three — The Harvard Children 141

Appendix Four — Seal Island Supplies 147

Paean To Harvard by Matron Mrs Ann Dalton 158

About The Author 159

Acknowledgements

This book would never have been written without the help and encouragement of Ralph Warner and his daughter, Valerie, who typed the manuscript. I also offer my sincere thanks to the following, who helped in so many different ways: Dr D. A. J. Tyrrell and Dr W. Craig for suggesting the book in the first place; my late wife, Gladys, for her help and understanding in my work at Harvard; my present wife, Kathleen, for her infinite patience; my two sons, David and Michael; Josephine and Desmond Buchanan for Diary and photographs of the Island Scheme; Miss T. Borthwick-Clarke; Dr G. I. Barrow; Dr P. Higgins; Mr A. Amos; Mr S. Hall; Mr and Mrs C. Aldridge; Mrs A. Rogers; Mrs P. Brown; Mrs M. Andrews; Mrs A. Dalton; Miss J. Dunning; Mr and Mrs M. Kernhert; Mrs Lois M. Simon; Mrs S. Rees; and Mrs F. Scott. Finally, a word of thanks to Dharmesh Gordon, of the Everyman Bookshop, Salisbury, for pointing me in the direction of Danny Howell, who very kindly agreed to publish this book.

K.R.T.

*To the thousands of volunteers
who have made it possible
to write this book*

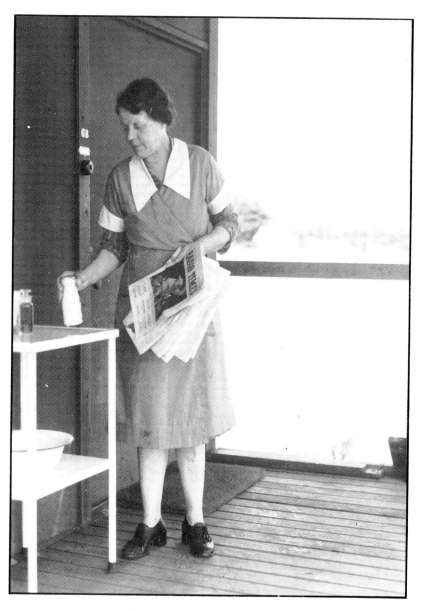

Leaving milk and the papers outside a volunteer's flat.

Preface

By Dr D. A. J. Tyrrell

C.B.E., M.D., D.S.E., F.R.C.P., F.R.C.PATH., F.R.S.

The Common Cold Research Unit was a unique institution —
the only place in the world where human beings were regularly
infected with respiratory viruses as part of a long term
programme of research on acute respiratory infections. At first
the work was directed at finding the viruses that caused colds,
and how to propagate and study them in the laboratory. The
laboratory techniques were developed and used throughout the
world. Later we studied how influenza viruses might be
attenuated to produce a vaccine strain, and whether it would be
possible to prevent or treat colds by giving antiviral drugs. We
also studied how viruses produced the signs and symptoms of
illness and possible methods of preventing this. This involved
detailed work on the importance of immunity and on
psychological factors and susceptibility to infection and illness.
In the last years we applied newer molecular techniques to
detecting and analyzing viruses and the response of the body to
them.

In all this work we regarded our volunteers as experimental
animals, or as units in a statistical analysis, as someone once
said "In answering these scientific questions one man equals
one mouse". Indeed, some volunteers fully understood this
and were really quite proud to think that they had appeared as a
dot on a graph on the pages of a scientific journal.

However, at the Salisbury Unit they were never "just" guinea
pigs. The reasons were partly philosophical — the volunteers
were our fellow human beings, to whom we related as people
and whom we treated as we would like to have been treated if
our roles had been reversed. However, our reasons were also

9

practical — if we didn't treat our volunteers well they wouldn't come and our experiments would not even get started.

The Unit was, I believe, a success in contributing steadily to the pool of knowledge, and being known and respected for this around the world. But that scientific success, which has been reported elsewhere, was only possible because of the skill and dedication with which volunteers were recruited and cared for throughout 44 years of continuous operation. This was possible partly because of a specially British response to the invitation to come and join in as partners in the research effort. But it was also the result of the mixture of charm and sensitivity, mixed with efficiency and strict discipline, with which volunteers were recruited and cared for at the Unit. Though it was so important, that mixture has never been described at length. There is no-one better fitted than "Tom" to tell that part of the story and I welcome the fact that he has taken so much trouble to gather many of the facts and incidents together and set them down on paper.

Foreword

The years teach much which the days never know
Ralph Waldo Emerson

The story of the Common Cold Research Unit at Salisbury, in Wiltshire, provides an example of ultimate success after a long period of apparent failure. From its inception in 1946 the primary aim of the Unit was to develop laboratory methods for the cultivation and identification of possible causative viruses, testing the experimentally produced materials for their capacity to give rise to colds by instilling small quantities into the noses of healthy volunteers. For more than twelve years no reliable method of cultivation could be found. A breakthrough occurred in 1959 and from then onwards discoveries came thick and fast, the laboratory rapidly gaining recognition as a leading centre of research into viruses of the respiratory tract. The Unit continued to attract volunteers for various investigations of the properties of such viruses until, having attained its principal objectives, it closed in 1989.

Situated at the top of a hill on the south-western outskirts of Salisbury, with open country and farmland beyond, the Common Cold Research Unit was well adapted to house healthy and active volunteers in relative isolation from other people, thereby reducing the risk of their coming into contact with natural sources of infection or of passing on experimentally-induced colds to members of the general public. Moreover, pre-existing accommodation, though originally designed for a somewhat different purpose, proved to be admirably suited to the needs of the research project. During the Second World War the site had been occupied by a field hospital,[1] formally opened in 1941 and later transferred to the control of the United States Army. The events that led to the establishment of this hospital and its subsequent contributions

11

to the study of epidemic diseases have been summarized by Sir Christopher Andrewes[2] and it will suffice here to state that the main buildings were pre-fabricated in America and shipped across the Atlantic. The professional and technical staff were also American.

After the war had ended the American Red Cross and Harvard Medical School, who had been the original sponsors of the hospital, presented the buildings and equipment to the British Ministry of Health, whose hope was that the facilities these offered might continue to be used for epidemiological studies. Dr C. H. Andrewes, who had been working on viruses for many years at the National Institute for Medical Research, saw in this American legacy a golden opportunity to extend investigations into the causation of the common cold. The lack of any animal, other than man and the higher apes, known to be susceptible to this infection implied the use of volunteers on a scale greater than any hitherto contemplated. Harvard Hospital provided just the accommodation needed for a continual flow of *human* guinea pigs prepared to live for short periods in reasonable attractive conditions involving an adequate degree of segregation without irksome confinement.

Thus it was that the Common Cold Research Unit came into being. It was a joint enterprise by the Medical Research Council, which employed the medical, laboratory and office staff, and the Ministry of Health, which engaged the catering and maintenance staff and the matron. During its existence the Unit attracted 20,000 volunteers, many of whom returned at regular intervals. In the early years the continuation of the work was threatened on several occasions for the lack of sufficiently encouraging results, but wise counsels prevailed and, in the long term, were vindicated.

The conduct of the scientific studies and their results have been recorded in the periodical medical literature and in separate publications by Sir Christopher Andrewes, Dr D. A. J. Tyrrell and others. These accounts have one feature in common. They have all been written, as it were, from Army Headquarters by those involved in the planning of the research; but there is another story to be told, from the standpoint of the

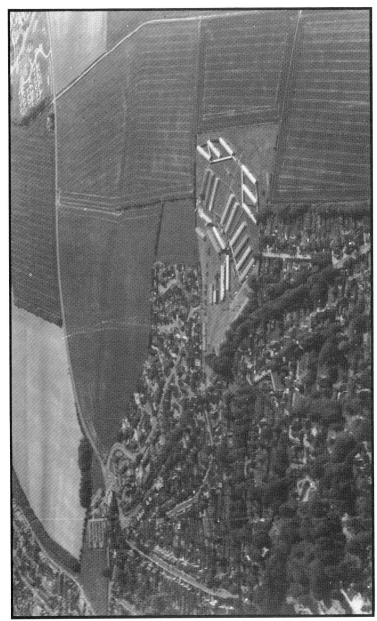

The Common Cold Research Unit (just right of the picture centre) in relation to Salisbury. The Bournemouth road is top left, and Odstock Hospital is top right.

troops in the field, the supporting staff and the volunteers themselves, whose co-operation was vital to the successful implementation of the plans. The two approaches are complementary and I know of no one better equipped to undertake the second of them than the author of this book. Keith Thompson, known affectionately to staff and volunteers alike as Tom, was present on the day when the very first group of volunteers arrived and remained on the staff until his retirement in 1982. He kept in touch with the Unit until it closed and he has given a vivid account of more than forty years of a unique episode in the history of medical research in Britain.

Dr A. T. Roden

M.D., D.P.H., D.C.H., F.F.C.M.

Medical Superintendent 1951–1956

References to Foreword

(1) The American Red Cross — Harvard Field Hospital Unit.
(2) Andrewes, Sir Christopher (1973). *In Pursuit of the Common Cold.* William Heinemann Medical Books Limited. London.

Introduction

During the First World War the Government of the United States of America asked the Harvard Medical School to organize Medical Service Units to enter the fighting area.

These Units arrived in Paris in April 1915 and served with the British Forces, transferring to the American Army when their country entered the War in 1917.

Less than ten days after the German invasion of Poland and the British declaration of War in September 1939, the Harvard Medical School once again met to decide what could be done to assist in the emergency existing in Britain and Europe.

The Harvard Medical School agreed after many meetings that its expertise in epidemic prevention, nutrition, sanitation and physiological treatment of shell shock would be the most helpful way in which it could be of value to Britain. Nothing much happened in the early months, (the "Phoney War" as it was known) until the evacuation of the British Forces at Dunkirk and the fall of France in July 1940, and it was at this time that Professor R. P. Linstead, an Englishman, who had been working at the Harvard Medical School returned home. He approached the British Government enquiring if they would be interested in the Harvard Medical School sending a medical group to assist with any of the services required from the specialized fields previously mentioned. The British Ministry of Health replied they would be deeply grateful, especially if such a mission could be supplemented by the provision of a hospital for such diseases. There was at that time a serious shortage of such hospitals in Britain. The manufacture of equipment for use by the armed forces made it almost impossible for us to provide and equip new hospitals .

The Harvard Medical School met to consider the request and decided that it was of the utmost importance to help. The decision had the full support of President Roosevelt and a cable was sent to the Minister of Health on 31 July 1940. The cable read, "Harvard ready to send advance group of experts, have given careful study to Hospital project, fund raising for any purpose very difficult,· would need some British financial support".

A return cable from the Ministry of Health on 2 August 1940 read, "Gratefully accept your generous offer, consultation desirable to answer your questions and development of future plans, cordially invite your advance party at your earliest convenience".

Harvard selected Dr John E. Gordon and Dr John R. Mote as the advance guard to England. Transport arrangements were most difficult at that time as passports were not being issued to American citizens to travel on belligerent ships, and being neutral, America had no ships plying between belligerent ports. The situation was, however, overcome with the help of the U.S. State Department.

The doctors landed in Liverpool on 15 August 1940 and moved to London where they remained during the most critical stages of the Battle of Britain. They were there on that crucial Friday 13 September 1940, when the bombing reached its peak and the British people were convinced that the air bombardment was a prelude to an armed invasion. One American correspondent commenting on the indiscriminant bombing of civilians as a new type of war referred to the British as "A hard pressed people standing in the breech of civilisation".

The Harvard Medical School went to work immediately seeking the help of many organizations for money. The Red Cross took constructive action in providing funds and the nursing and non-professional staff for a 125 bed hospital. The buildings, personnel and equipment had to be shipped to England, with the constant threat of losses by enemy action at sea and danger of death from the air for Harvard personnel already in London. Another difficulty the Harvard Medical School encountered was criticism in their own country against such a project, regarding it as "an emotional jaunt," providing no sound scientific research, and not related to American problems in their own public health services.

In April 1941 came the first harsh reminder that the main venture was no tea party, but a serious life and death affair. News arrived in America that Dr John E. Gordon and Dr Paul B. Beeson the advance consultants, had been blown across their rooms and cut by flying glass when their lodgings in London were destroyed by a bomb during an air raid. Two months later as a result of a ship being torpedoed five Red Cross nurses were lost. Several others spent 19 days in open boats to be finally landed in Iceland and Northern Ireland, some so badly exhausted and shocked they were invalided home.

After many setbacks the Hospital arrived in this country and was erected on its present site, being formally opened on 22 September 1941. Why was the site of Salisbury chosen? I believe (remember I am not a scientist) that it was ideal for the epidemiological studies, the site was near the Southern Command H.Q. should military help be needed, also near the city of Salisbury for supplies and rail communication, as well as easily being available if needed during treatment of highly infectious diseases. For the first 20 months the 125 beds received both civilian and military patients suffering from communicable diseases. When America entered the War on 15 July 1942, Harvard passed into the hands of the United States Army, and played an important part in the American war effort.

Additional buildings were erected to house technicians, to provide a training school and to extend laboratories. Harvard became the main blood transfusion centre for the forces in Britain and Europe.

By the end of the War in June 1945, 20 additional buildings had been added to the original 22 sent over five years earlier. Harvard had made a name for itself in the study of communicable diseases.

The American personnel eventually evacuated Harvard in Autumn 1945, leaving it in immaculate condition. A platoon of British Army personnel moved in as caretakers.

As mentioned the Ministry of Health (now the D.H.S.S.) played a major part in bringing Harvard to England, the Medical Research Council also being involved with the war time study of epidemiology. What would Harvard be used for now that the war was over? There were political and sentimental aspects to be considered, plus the scientific reputation and the cordiality between America and Britain and more important between Harvard University, its Faculty of Medicine, the Ministry of Health and the Medical Research Council. It was Dr W. H. Bradley from the Ministry of Health who played the key rôle in the building of Harvard at Salisbury, who suggested it should be used for the common cold investigation. The layout of its buildings made it easy for adaption to research into the common cold, and a continuation of its war time rôle — the study of communicable diseases. Research into the cause of the common cold had begun pre-war by Sir Christopher Andrewes, who discovered that human volunteers were needed if he was to have any success.

The first human volunteers were not used until 1931 when Sir Christopher Andrewes enrolled students from St Bartholomew's Hospital. He explained to them that as he could not get chimpanzees, he considered the next best thing would be a "Barts" student. He promised that he would not do as his friend Dr Dochez had done, who being curious to know what the chimps did after the scientist had left decided to peep through the keyhole only to be greeted by the eye of an equally curious chimp obviously with the same thought in mind with regard to the scientist on his departure from the laboratory.

Joining The Unit

After being demobilised from the Services in April 1946, I obtained work as a driver to the Medical Council at their laboratories in Hollyhill, Hampstead, London, being virtually next door to my parents' home. I got the job on the understanding that I went to Harvard Hospital, Salisbury, Wiltshire, where research into the common cold was to take place. I was informed that I would be returning to Hampstead in approximately three years, the time it would take to glean the information on viruses causing the common cold.

I arrived at Harvard on Monday 16 June 1946 and was immediately confronted by two contrasts. Firstly, a conglomeration of huts painted in drab war time camouflage

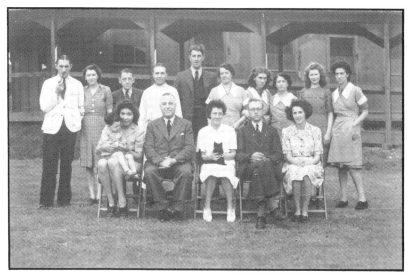

All 15 members of staff pictured a few days before the First Trial.

19

guarded it seemed by two black towers, a sight I did not appreciate. Secondly, these buildings overlooked on three sides the beautiful panoramic views of the Wiltshire countryside with the Hampshire Avon and the small Ebble trout stream flowing past the picturesque villages of Nunton, Odstock and Homington, and the rolling hills sloping down to the Chalke Valley.

My personal thoughts on viewing this glorious countryside were of how lucky I was to be in such delightful surroundings. This, I suppose is why I stayed at Harvard until my retirement in 1982.

As for the drabness of the buildings, these were later painted in colours to blend in with the surrounding countryside. I am certain that the surrounding landscape of hills, woods and rivers was a major reason why the recruitment of volunteers was so successful, especially those living and working in big cities.

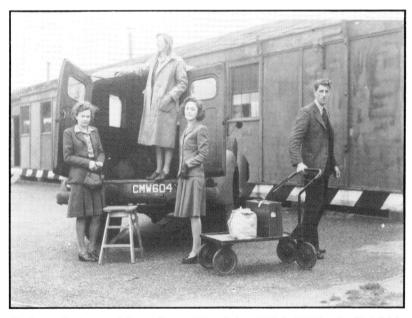

Student volunteers arriving at Harvard Hospital on 17 July 1946 for the First Trial.

Preparation For The First Trial

The following day, 17 June 1946, I met Dr D. M. Chalmers the Unit's Medical Superintendant who outlined the common cold experiment and the need for volunteers and the part they would play in the successful study of the cold virus, and that without them the Unit could not function.

It was from these early days that all members of staff became aware that the volunteers were to be treated as V.I.P.'s. Dr Chalmers then explained that the study of the common cold virus in co-operation with the volunteers would be in the form of 10 day periods called Trials.

These Trials would commence on Wednesday, volunteers' Intake Day, finishing on the Saturday week, when the volunteers went home. Further details of volunteer trials and the isolation procedure will be given in later chapters.

The first Trial was to start on Wednesday 17 July 1946, which was only four weeks away. What a daunting task. There was much to do.

One small incident I remember at this time was with my ration book. I purchased my week's allowance of meat, butter and sugar at the butcher's and corner shop in the local village of Harnham. My 4oz of chop disappeared before my eyes as I proceeded to cook it on the overheated oil fired stove in the Unit's kitchen. Another meatless week!

Dr Chalmers, an excellent Administrator and organiser, had already worked out detailed routines for dealing with the volunteers. These were much the same 40 years on. The immediate priorities laid out by Dr Chalmers were:—

1. Set up an administration office
2. Engagement of office staff — a temporary secretary had already arrived from the Medical Research Council at Hampstead

3. Prepare volunteer accommodation
4. Appointment of general staff
5. Prepare staff living quarters
6. Set up a temporary laboratory, later to be known as LAB.3

We did not use the same Administration Office as the Americans. This was a Nissen building and not within the administration structure of the Common Cold Unit.

With the help of our temporary typist, the room which was to become the Administration Office was cleared of paper and empty animal cages. This room and others adjoining it had been used as pathology laboratories.

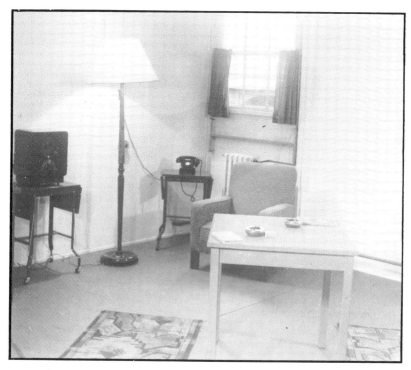

Volunteers' sitting room, ready and waiting for its first occupants.

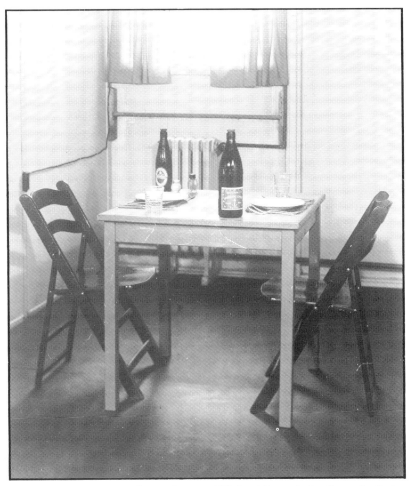

Table and chairs in one of the volunteers' kitchen/diners during the early days.

We were now in business. The typewriter "clicked" away with letters going out to the local papers advertising for a cook, kitchen assistant, general domestics, a porter, and other staff.

Within a day or so Miss Irene Newlands, the Unit's first permanent Secretary arrived, and on her heels, Miss Barbara Rae, taking up the post of Matron.

23

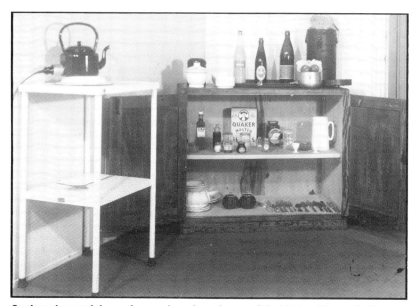

Cupboard, containing rations and crockery, in one of the kitchen/diners. Notice the fly swot on the lower shelf of the table.

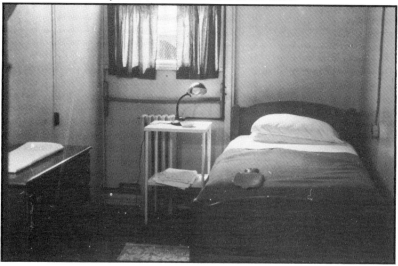

Volunteers' all-American equipped bedroom, complete with furniture, bed linen, bedside-lamp, and hot-water bottle.

Right: Each volunteer's flat had its own gowns worn by doctors and scientists when entering. The stirrup-pump, a wartime fire precaution, hangs on the wall ready for use.

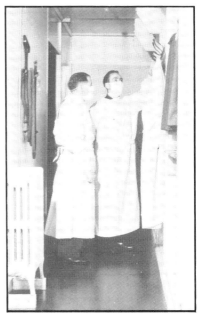

Below: Delivering food containers during the early trials. The outside handwashing facilities, which included an enamel bowl, can be seen.

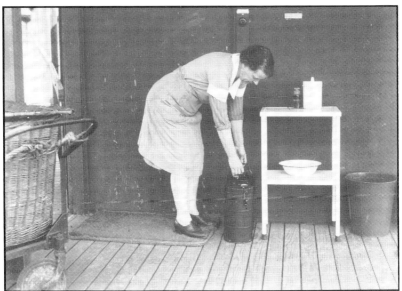

Time was short and there was so much to do. Everything needed to furnish volunteer and staff accommodation, kitchen, dining room and office, with the exception of the typewriter was on site — all left by the Americans. It needed to be put in place, cleaned and polished. There were also 400 war time "Blackout" curtains to be taken down.

Contractors had now been employed to carry out such work as re-positioning of walkways and partitioning the interiors of each building to be used for living acommodation. A certain amount of plumbing needed to be done. The Office switchboard was installed — thank goodness — with extensions to all volunteer flats, kitchen, dining room and laboratory. This made life much easier — no more blowing a whistle when someone was wanted on the one and only telephone.

With a week before the first volunteers arrival all the required staff had been employed — including the Unit's chef, Mr Cameron Clarke, a most important person. Food rationing was still in force, therefore his job was to make the most of it, as well as providing enough to keep the volunteers happy. He was given accommodation on site. The office staff increased to two with the arrival of Miss Priscilla Newman, our switchboard operator and typist.

Wednesday 17 July arrived, everything for the first intake was as ready as it ever would be. Looking back, much would not be accepted today. The redeeming features then were the comfortable living quarters, continuous hot water and central heating, with cooked breakfast, lunch and evening meal delivered to the door, plus no queueing for the weekly rations. Washing up facilities were rather primitive, being done in the bathroom wash-hand basin. The facility for the daily visits of doctors and scientists to wash their hands before medical examination was, done outside the flat entrance door, in an enamel bowl before entry. This was, of course soon changed. Had it been in force during the coming 1946/47 severe winter, the bowls would have become a mould for "Ice Discus".

Recruiting Of Volunteers

Recruitment for volunteers was extended beyond St Bartholomew's Hospital. Prior to the first Trial at Harvard Sir Christopher Andrewes and Dr Chalmers visited the universities explaining to students the need for volunteers and how they could help with research into the common cold and at the same time continue their studies during their vacation. They emphasized that all travelling expenses would be paid and all meals supplied. Comfortable accommodation would be provided and the number one attraction which always encouraged people to volunteer was the delightful countryside that surrounds Harvard, for walks with flat mates without braking the isolation procedure.

The first Trial consisted of 12 volunteers followed by five all student Trials. We could rely on students during their Christmas, Easter and summer vacations only. The common cold research programme however needed a continuous flow of volunteers. Dr Chalmers and Mr Langford, the Administrator of Harvard Hospital, visited the W.D & H.O. Wills cigarette factory in Bristol, Imperial Chemical Industries (ICI), and the British Red Cross Society as part of their recruitment drive and were delighted when these organisations permitted their staff to participate in the Trials on full pay. There were now sufficient volunteers to go through until the 1946 Christmas university vacation.

With the current anti-smoking publicity the media would have a field day with headlines such as "Medical Research Use Tobacco Barons To Study Viruses." However it was at the time that the media became interested with such headlines as "Britain Wins War, Now Fights The Common Cold." The press were invited to Salisbury, and Harvard held its first press conference with 40 journalists being given a talk by Sir Christopher Andrewes during which he emphasized the importance of acquiring volunteers, and how the press could help by giving the project news space. He explained how the volunteers were housed together in pairs. (He wrote in his book *The Pursuit Of The Common Cold* that a little devil caused him to say entirely on the spur of the moment that it might suit honeymoon couples. Journalists ears pricked up and rushed notes were made on pads with the resulting national press coverage describing Harvard as the place for honeymooners to go. "Free Honeymoon Hotel").

Such press comments were not good for the Harvard image, which, of course, was the serious study of a common virus. We were inundated with enquiries, receiving over 2,000 letters. Although further press conferences were held in later years they never generated the same impact. The Central Office Of Information became interested and made a 20 minute film during January 1947 — a very bad winter with freezing/icy conditions which meant that yards of the film unit's cabling became frozen to the wooden walkways. My future wife and I were taking the part of volunteers and were supposed to look warm and cheerful, enjoying ourselves — very difficult in the circumstances.

In later years I learned from a close Army friend who lived in a small Welsh village that it caused a minor disaster in his household when he watched the film on television during the family's evening meal.

Recognizing me he shouted "It's Tom, it's Tom," and jumping up from the table pulled the cloth and table contents to the floor!

In February 1947, as a result of the press coverage, we had our first cross-section of the general public taking part in Trials, i.e housewives, a coal miner, a bus driver and secretaries, in fact people from all walks of life began to give us a continuous intake of volunteers, especially during the summer months. Naturally the numbers fell during the winter. Dr Hill, later to become Lord Hill, known as the Radio Doctor was very successful in recruiting volunteers when he mentioned our needs in his five minute morning radio programme.

Fortunately the press, radio and television became interested

Would you like
TEN DAYS FREE HOLIDAY
and Travel Expenses paid?

All you have to do is to help the research into the common cold and influenza at the Research Centre in Salisbury, Wilts.

Over 400 people come every year but MORE ARE WANTED URGENTLY.

Comfortable accommodation for married or single people aged 18-50 years.

If interested write for details to:
COMMON COLD UNIT, SALISBURY, WILTS SP2 8BW
or phone 0722 22485 between 9 a.m. and 5 p.m.

A publicity hand-out, offering a free holiday and travel expenses to would-be volunteers.

in winter flu's and colds, giving good news coverage to epidemics which broke out in various parts of the world. Harvard was continually contacted for information relating to each outbreak. As a result of which the Harvard scientists were interviewed by such personalities as Dr Bronowski, Lady Barnett, Raymond Baxter, Richard Dimbleby and the BBC Science Correspondent.

From time to time Harvard Scientists appeared on television interviewed by news-presenters and if given a chance would mention the need for volunteers. We also had visits from correspondents of various women's magazines and other publications. Correspondents usually visited Harvard on the Thursday when isolation had finished and volunteers were free to be interviewed, it was also possible for photographs to be

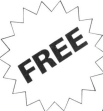

A 10 DAY HOLIDAY
AT ANY TIME OF YEAR

YES, comfortable accommodation in centrally heated flats, three cooked meals a day, £1₂5 a day pocket-money, and the cost of your return rail or coach fare to Salisbury from any place south of a line from Glasgow to Edinburgh – All that in lovely Wiltshire countryside with facilities for those who like an active life and for those who want to relax.

Does it sound too good to be true? Well you must be between 18 and 50 years of age and in good health, and you must be willing to have a drop put in each nostril. These drops which may contain a virus cause a mild cold in one volunteer in three. Most volunteers consider this a small price to pay for a holiday which is otherwise free, and many make return visits annually.

Volunteers are housed in flats, either married couples or in twos or threes of the same sex. Each flat has a living room with TV and radio, a kitchenette, bathroom and either two or three bedrooms. Some volunteers come with a friend, but others like to share a flat with a companion with similar interests. Many new friendships have been formed from a visit to the Common Cold Research Unit.

All staff – medical, nursing, administrative, catering and domestic are friendly and helpful to volunteers and try to make the holiday enjoyable. There are facilities for reading and relaxing as well as for indoor and outdoor games and walking, but you are free to choose. Continued research into cause, prevention and cure of colds depends on the participation and co-operation of volunteers prepared to come to Salisbury for a period of 10 days. If you would like to help the community and at the same time enjoy a novel holiday please send for an application form and detailed information to:

COMMON COLD UNIT, HARVARD HOSPITAL, COOMBE ROAD,
SALISBURY, WILTS SP2 8BW

**Publicity pamphlet given to volunteers on their departure, for them to fix on works'
or office notice-boards.**

taken of the Unit, i.e. laboratories, kitchen, games rooms, volunteers' accommodation and even volunteers receiving their "pocket money" (to be mentioned in further chapters).

A good intake of volunteers continued through the 1950s and early 60s by students, returned visits, recommendations by satisfied volunteers, articles in magazines, local newspapers, talks by members of staff to groups of people in colleges, womens institutes etc. By the late 1960s we started to advertise in a mild way. We had a request for a volunteer's leaflet to be printed. These were handed to volunteers as they left for display on notice boards in their place of work, at the same time they were sent to local libraries, council offices and hospitals. Harvard was always well supported by members of the nursing profession.

By 1975 we took a more direct line of advertising for volunteers, care was taken not to attract people who expected a "Holiday Camp" atmosphere, with no understanding of the isolation procedure. With careful wording and using the right papers and journals it met with some success. Harvard and its need for volunteers was now becoming perhaps, not a household word, but very well known, so advertising prompted people to come. As many said on arrival, they had always thought of coming but seeing the advertisement had inspired them to do something about it.

For many reasons we were not getting the same student response as in previous years and it was dicided that I should visit the universities within reach in the spring and autumn of each year. Talking to the Student Union officials and encouraging them to place the need for volunteers in their news sheets, mentioning, as Sir Christopher Andrewes and Dr Chalmers had done in the beginning, the opportunities for study, comfortable accommodation, good food free travel and pocket money.

With 40 years behind us many people were coming each year. Groups of volunteers, who without breaking the isolation procedure had become friends and arranged to return in following years, with no less than six from one family returning for many years.

By an odd coincidence this very day as I write on volunteer recruitment, Dr P. Higgins, a member of the scientific research team, along with two volunteers on their ninth visit to Harvard were interviewed by the BBC/Television news presenters. Dr Higgins explained the need for more volunteers and the two volunteers telling how pleasant it was to have taken part in nine trials, and how they would be willing to come again.

However with the prompting of the media, advertising etc., a steady flow of volunteers was maintained.

From Small Beginnings

When the Unit opened in 1946 it began with only 12 full and two part time members of staff consisting of the medical superintendant, administration officer, matron, one laboratory technician, chef, second cook, two kitchen assistants, kitchen porter, two cleaning ladies (one full and one part time), general porter, part time linen room lady and myself as driver/handyman and general "dogs body" spending most of my time putting up shelves and other odd jobs in the office, kitchen or wherever required.

The laboratory technician, Mr A. Lane, was on loan from MRC Laboratories, Hampstead. His laboratory at Harvard consisted of one room in the administration building, indentified as "LAB no. 3." This room had been used during the War as the Hospital mortuary, and still housed the mortuary slab and washing facilities, all in working order. The slab was covered with ply wood enabling it to be used as a laboratory work bench. There are few research units that can boast of this dual rôle!

In the autumn of 1946 Mr Langford the temporary Administrative Officer, left taking a post within his profession as a dentist. Mr Alan Waltho followed and soon after his arrival it was decided to transfer the Common Cold Laboratory from Hampstead, opening up our own laboratories at Harvard.

We used the building parallel to the Administrative Office, known as "LAB no. 2." The Unit now had its own scientific staff. Dr K. R. Dumbell and Dr E. J. R. Lowbury plus laboratory technicians and part time workers for glassware cleaning and sterilizing. With the opening of this laboratory the Unit became alive, in addition to more staff there were many interesting visitors. This new impetus was the beginning of Harvard's recognition as a leading research centre for viruses of the respiratory tract.

Early in 1947 Mr Bunce and his assistant were employed as groundsmen, the grass having previously been cut by the next door farmer with his horsedrawn cutter. The only mechanical mower we had was one left by the Americans and repaired in our workshops. New ones were in very short supply.

The kitchen staff was increased when the dining room was opened for staff lunches and evening meals, the later lasting for only a few months. A bar was opened for the sale of alcoholic and soft drinks, trusting people to enter in a book drinks taken and their cost. This facility was short lived, not much from dishonesty, more from forgetfulness.

In 1948 an Air Hygiene Unit moved down to Salisbury from Hampstead, they used the building indentified as "LAB no. 4." This was of great interest to me liking anything mechanical, for they had metal milling machines, lathes, drills etc. The Unit was staffed by Dr Owen Lidwell and Dr James Lovelock plus two assistants. They were to be the start of a second laboratory which a few years later became a thriving concern housing a department of the World Health Organization.

Around this time we started a sports club with both football and cricket teams. Every able-bodied male member of staff had to play to make up the 11 for football. We played about six matches for one season only, winning just one game, but it was great fun. Harvard had no home ground and always played away, travelling on bicycles. In the summer the neighbouring farmer allowed us to use one of his fields for cricket.

The number of staff grew with six families living in the staff accommodation creating a friendly fraternity which although the volunteers were in isolation brought them into this community atmosphere, they did not feel so isolated after working hours, when daily staff had left for home, a friendly "Hello, how are you?" could always be exchanged. On the other side of the coin, with staff coming and going, volunteers were less likely to come into close contact with one another thereby breaking isolation.

The last department to open was Harvard's Animal House. The same building the Americans had used for that purpose. There was never any intensive experiments using animals, a

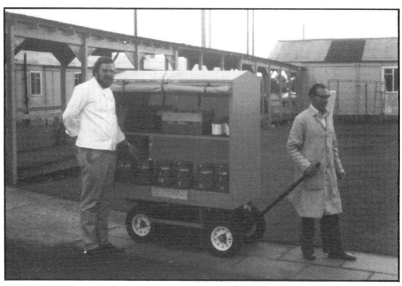

Meals being delivered at Harvard Hospital during 1978.

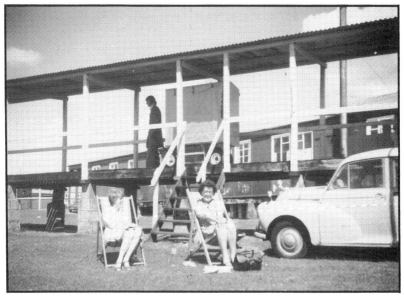

Two volunteers enjoying the sun while waiting for their meal (1970s).

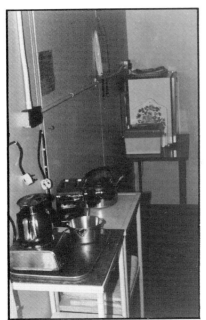 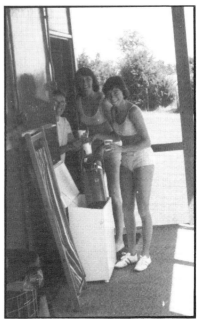

Stainless steel utensils in the modernised rooms.

Flatmates collecting their lunch outside their door after the meal trolley had departed (1978).

few guinea pigs and rabbits only. They were mainly used for taking a few drops of blood. In many ways they were pets, especially with the children, and lived to an old age. The Animal House if only part time, completed the basic staff compliment. Naturally, as the scientific work intensified so the number of staff increased, from the beginning with 14 to, at its height in the 1960s, 28 full time and 10 part time members.

A mention must be made of departments and people who staffed them. Of course one department relies on another for the smooth running of a unit and this never more so than at Harvard. Dealing with members of the public volunteering to be given cold or flu viruses, their well being was of utmost importance.

The office is where the first contact is made and very often an opinion is formed. Harvard was always on the look out for

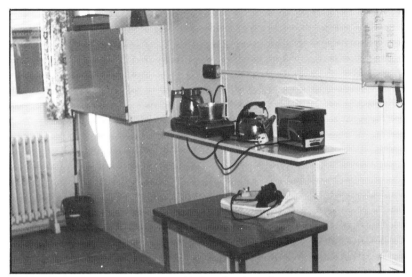

A much updated kitchen for the volunteers.

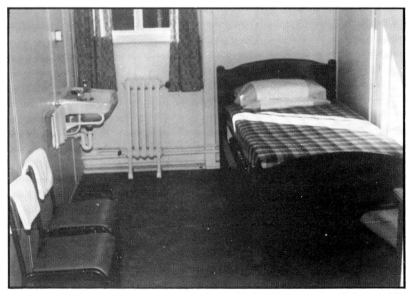

A basin with hot and cold running water in the Medical Room replaced the outside bowl for hand-washing.

volunteers and tried to employ office staff with a good personality, especially its switchboard operator. The first as previously mentioned, was Miss Priscilla Newman who later became responsible for the whole office. Two of her sisters succeeded her with telephone duties. Office girls come and go, usually marrying and starting a family. However, we were lucky in employing Miss Angela Bundy in 1952, she became Mrs Sims, marrying in 1957 and remained in the office until the Unit's closure. Angela knew the answer to any query, carrying out an immaculate job as a paymistress to the volunteers and staff, checking all invoices and accounts, writing out cheques for signature and payment. Angela was also the Harvard detective. A few volunteers when over the age limit and hoping to continue their visits took to changing their names, using false addresses and lowering their ages. Angela would always detect something in their application form that made her suspicious, usually their handwriting. On one occasion when giving a lady the benefit of the doubt she arrived having dyed her hair,

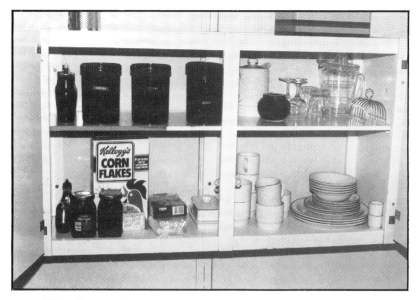

Wine glasses and Poole pottery feature in the volunteers' cupboard.

wearing dark glasses and a change of accent, unfortunately for her she was not a very good actress!

Volunteers, who came alone, were usually housed in twos or threes. These pairings being done by the office staff, comparing the application forms for age, occupation, hobbies etc. They became very good at this, very few were unable to get along, some finding new friends and arranging to meet up again at Harvard the following year or even years later.

Although the "Computer Age" came to the Harvard Office, staff did not lose their personal and friendly approach. Miss Teresa Borthwick-Clarke now working with Angela has been most helpful to me in the research of this attempt to document something of the Harvard scene.

Many volunteers fell in love with the Wiltshire countryside, selling up and buying homes in the Salisbury area.

Reading the many verses the volunteers have written and their praise to the catering and office staff, especially appreciation for their shopping trips as isolation did not allow

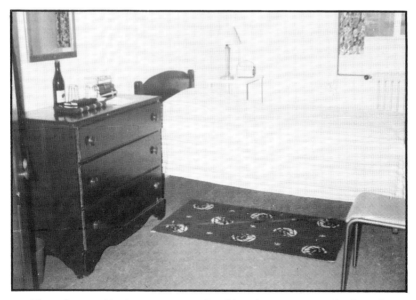

The volunteers' bedrooms were updated but the carpets remained small.

39

volunteers to shop for themselves. Harvard had a system whereby once they had settled into their flats there were two lists to be filled in, one for library and indoor games, the other for shopping requirements. These were placed in the internal post box and collected the morning following the "intake day." The library and games requests were dealt with by matron and the shopping by the office, Angela giving Mrs Audrey Rogers cash for their shopping needs. Volunteers were requested, where at all possible, to enter the bulk of their requirements on this list to last for the whole of the trial. There could not be a hard and fast rule and further shopping was carried out daily, with the cost being deducted from the volunteers' "pocket money."

Harvard's Directors

Harvard's first monetary grant was for a three year period, after which only a one year grant was given, then two years extending to four, five or six years, eventually adding up to 43 years of grant aid.

The prominent staff members responsible for obtaining these grants were its three directors, beginning with the one who started the Common Cold Project, Sir Christopher Andrewes, who lived to the ripe age of 92 in the nearby village of Coombe Bissett.

I remember his arrival during the first trial with the late Lady Andrewes and their three teenage sons in his 1934 12 hp Austin Open Tourer, and alighting from the car with his butterfly net in one hand and jar in the other. Sir Christopher, being a keen entomologist, wasted no time in hunting for new specimens for his collection.

As its Director, Sir Christopher visited Harvard for a few days during each trial. He worked mainly at the Institute of Medical Research in Mill Hill and being an eminent virologist he travelled worldwide.

Prior to his retirement in 1961 he discussed with me the possibility of finding a plot of land on which he could build a bungalow. I was fortunate in finding an ideal plot only two miles from Harvard, situated on a hillside overlooking the village of Coombe Bissett and surrounding countryside with the village church in the foreground. For him and Lady Andrewes it was ideal, enabling him to continue with his entomological studies. A very interesting BBC/TV broadcast on the subject was made from his home.

Following his retirement in 1961 the Directorship of Harvard was taken by Dr Alick Isaacs. He was very well liked by all the Harvard staff, being a friendly and happy person of a generous disposition. Unfortunately he died in January 1967 at the early age of 45, never having been resident at the Unit.

Dr Isaacs with his Swiss co-worker Dr J. Lindenmann discovered Interferon, a substance the body produces to prevent secondary infection.

Dr D. A. J. Tyrrell followed Dr Isaacs and remained in the post until the Unit's closure. He joined and became resident at the Unit in 1957, arriving with Mrs Tyrrell and their two daughters, Frances aged six, Susan, four and three year old son, Stephen. They had journeyed down from Sheffield in their 1956 Austin A30. The ladened roof rack made the car resemble the Eiffel Tower on wheels. They were a happy family who easily fitted into the Harvard scene. Dr Tyrrell was a tireless worker approaching his subject with determination. The contributions made by these three men in scientific research will likely be commented upon in the future by medical historians.

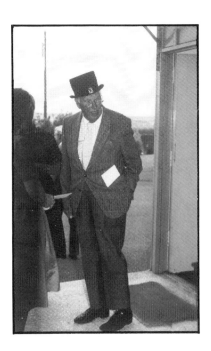

Sir Christopher Andrewes, in topper, on his 90th birthday.

The Unit's Ten Medical Superintendents

The Harvard staff whatever their position, scientist or porter, have always worked as one to maintain a close and harmonious atmosphere with the volunteers. During the 43 years of the trials 20,000 volunteers were recruited, many returning time and time again — the "die-hards" returning annually. This close relationship and goodwill was a great help in recruiting volunteers, ensuring that they were well looked after on arrival. The Medical Superintendent was in the forefront of this responsibility. The general administration of the Unit was dealt with by him co-ordinating volunteer correspondence and recruitment with an interview with each on arrival prior to a medical examination before beginning the trial.

It was important that the people used in the common cold trials should be in good health, both for their sakes and also the Unit's. People suffering from an infection could be harmed by experimental procedures. The Medical Superintendent visited the volunteers each morning throughout the trial noting any symptoms which they may have developed from nasal drops given by the scientists. At the end of each trial he wrote a complete report on each volunteer. It was common for Medical Superintendents to carry out clinical studies of their own.

Dr T Sommerville followed Dr Chalmers after the latter's death in 1947. Dr Sommerville lived on site with his wife and three young daughters. He started the epidemiological studies in the Chalke Valley and also the island experiment. These experiments will be described in later chapters. Dr Sommerville was also an authority on malaria.

In 1951 Dr Sommerville moved to St Andrews in Scotland, his position being taken by Dr A. T. Roden who maintained his house in London, staying at Harvard during the trial periods.

Dr Roden continued the Chalke Valley Studies as well as being involved with other clinical studies. Dr Roden retired from Harvard in 1956.

Dr T. W. Field became the Unit's fourth Medical Superintendent, retaining his home in the Ross Valley — a delightful place which my family and I often visited. He stayed at Harvard with Mrs Field during the trials. Dr Field had been a Senior Medical Officer in Malaya and whilst at Harvard spent some time revising his book on malaria.

With the retirement of Dr Field in 1957 came Dr M. L. Bynoe, also an ex-Malayan Medical Officer. To start with Dr Bynoe lived at Harvard and then moved to Burley in the New Forest. Finding that to be too distant he moved back to the Salisbury area.

Dr and Mrs Bynoe had one son, Christopher, who became a Fleet Air Arm pilot. Tragically he was killed immediately after take off from HMS *Hermes* near Singapore.

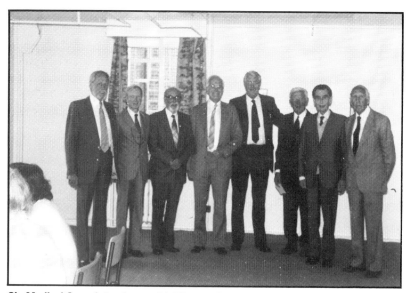

Six Medical Superintendents with Director Dr Tyrrell and Keith Thompson. Left to right: Dr Willman, Dr Barrow, Dr Wallace, Dr Tyrrell, Mr Thompson, Dr Hall, Dr Roden, and Dr Craig.

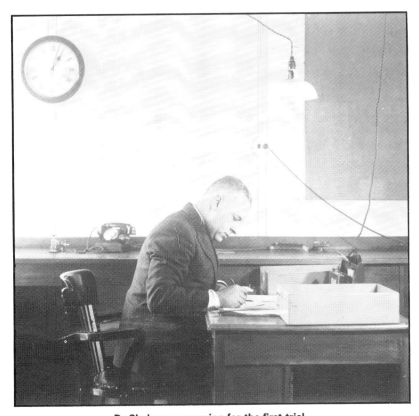

Dr Chalmers preparing for the first trial.

It was Dr Bynoe who suggested in 1961 that I should move from my position of driver and general workshop duties to the office taking on administrative work. This I did and under his guidance gradually took on more and more responsibilities, eventually taking a full administrative rôle. Mr C. Crabb, known to all as Cyril, carried on conscientiously with my late duties.

Dr Bynoe died of cancer in St George's Hospital, London, in June 1969 and I became very much more involved with events from that time. Before driving him to St George's he handed me a note giving me instructions for bringing his body back to

45

Salisbury and registering his death at Caxton Hall Registrar's Office, which I did with great difficulty after office hours. Also to help Mrs Bynoe to find suitable accommodation. During lunch on the way to the hospital he passed the comment that "This was the last meal of a condemned man."

Dr Field, Dr Bynoe and Miss E. Bullock, matron at that time, had all been prisoners of war of the Japanese and consequently suffered ill health as a result of the inhumane treatment they had received from their captors.

Dr T. Hall followed Dr Bynoe, living on site with his wife. He was a meticulous man who communicated well with the volunteers.

When Dr Hall retired in July 1973 the post was filled by Dr Wallace Craig, a retired heart consultant from the Whittington Hospital, Highgate, London. He and Mrs Craig, a distant relative of Lord Nelson, lived first at Harvard and then moved to a house overlooking the Harvard grounds. Dr Craig, very adept at communicating with the volunteers, was responsible for maintaining a high intake. He instilled an even friendlier atmosphere between volunteers and staff, especially during the intake day lunch and introductory talk. The formal classroom style of rows of volunteers and the speaker at the front was replaced by an informal loose circle with the speaker sitting among the volunteers, which made them feel even more at home. Dr Craig retired in September 1979.

In October 1979 Dr J. Wallace, residing at Harvard, became the Unit's eighth Medical Superintendent having retired from a senior post in the Scottish Blood Transfusion Service. He had helped to set up the Harvard Blood Bank used by the Armed Forces in Britain and Europe, especially during the Normandy landings.

It was while Dr Wallace was the Medical Superintendent that I retired in July 1982, he himself retiring in September of that year. Dr J. S. Willman followed, whom I have met on many occasions. He retired in November 1985.

Harvard's tenth and sadly last Medical Superintendent was to be Dr G. I. Barrow, no stranger to Harvard, having made numerous visits during earlier years.

Matrons Of Harvard

A female member of the nursing profession played an important part in the Harvard staff structure. She not only needed to be a qualified S.R.N. but also to have an understanding of human emotions. A mother confessor figure to volunteers and staff alike.

Although not as in the hospital sense responsible for a ward of nurses, she commanded the title of matron for her position and was someone for the volunteers to rely on for their clinical and welfare needs. Matron provided support to the Medical Superintendent and other medical staff in the provision of the health and welfare service to the volunteers. Also to assist in the organization and administration of the trials and in the selection of future volunteers. She co-operated with the Executive Officer in the general welfare of the volunteers and staff under her control, also for the kitchen, the chef and his staff and checking the weekly menus. On the matter of food supplies she worked closely with the Executive Officer, since the quantity and quality of food which the volunteers received was of the utmost importance.

Being in isolation and unable to shop for themselves, palatable meals for the volunteers was perhaps looked forward to more than anything else. She was also responsible for all the other domestic staff, their holiday and duty rosters, cleaning of volunteers' and staff quarters, the linen room and its supplies and inventory. In 1984 these duties were passed over to the Executive Officer.

She was, with the exception of one day off in the trial period, on hand at all times should a volunteer need her services. Eight of the Unit's ten matrons were unmarried, the other two living on site with their families. In the early years matron visited the volunteers with the Medical Superintendent on his morning round only. As trials became more complex it was necessary to

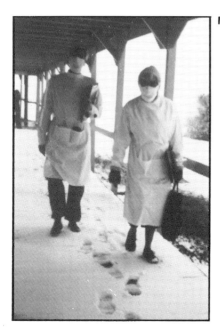

Matron Margaret Andrews (right) on her morning round with Dr Willman.

visit again in the early evening. Should Matron be wanted out of hours when the switchboard was closed her flat was easily identified by a garden watering can painted red. Why red? Previously some wag had placed several cans on as many doorsteps!

Matron presented the introductory talk to the volunteers at the beginning of each trial, explaining the routine and how to make the best of their stay, especially of country walks.

Each volunteer flat had its own medical room equipped with thermometers (one for each volunteer), examination couch etc. Her own clinical room which was used by the Medical Superintendent for a medical examination of each volunteer before taking part in the trial also included a drugs cabinet, all of which were under her care. Matron organized the volunteers' chest X-Rays which for the first 15 years of the trials took place at Harvard. The Americans had left excellent facilities which were used until spares became exhausted, after which she accompanied the volunteers to the local hospital.

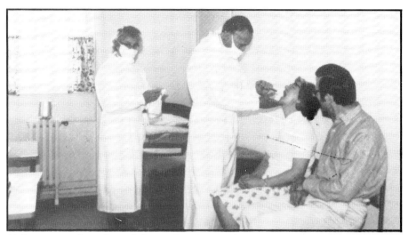

Volunteers undergoing a daily medical in one of the flats with Dr Craig and Matron Andrews.

Further duties included urine tests, instructing the volunteers in the use of thermometers and taking their own temperatures when required. When tissues supplied by the laboratory were used they had to be placed in a small plastic bag — five tissues to a bag — which were then returned to the laboratory for analysis. Mrs M. Andrews was the last Matron to carry out these duties and since her retirement in 1984 two nursing officers have shared these duties.

Miss B. Rae was the first matron. She was an ex-Service Nursing Officer who stayed for six months. Miss M. Gamble followed for a further year. Miss J. Macdonald who came from Scotland held the post for 12 years. She is remembered with affection having played a large part in giving the Unit its identity. Respected by volunteers and the Chalke Valley villagers alike for she made door to door calls in connection with the Chalke Valley epidemiology studies.

Miss E. Bullock was another long serving matron staying at Harvard for seven years after Miss MacDonald's retirement. It was not long after Miss Bullock's arrival that I transferred to my new job in administration. She gave me great help and support at that time. Sadly she died not long after retirement in April

1967 as a result of the ill-treatment she received in a Japanese prisoner of war camp during World War Two.

Miss M. Turnbull, the instigator of the watering can identification came next and stayed just two years. She was followed by Miss J. Bailey who had been a Nursing Officer at the Star and Garter Home for Disabled Servicemen, where she is now its matron. Miss J. Bowden was matron between 1972—1975.

To date matrons had always come from other parts of the country and it was thought that local appointments would encourage a longer stay than just two or three years. We were successful in appointing Mrs M. Andrews who was given on-site accommodation for her husband and three sons. Besides the nursing qualifications she had a friendly and motherly nature, someone the volunteers trusted on sight.

When finance became available Mrs Andrews and her linen room assistant, Mrs A. Rogers carried out a programme of upgrading the volunteers' accommodation. They replaced worn and drab curtains, bedspreads and tablecloths with more colourful and matching designs; this included sitting room, bedroom and bedside lampshades. The kitchen took on a new look with the substitution of ministry crockery for Poole pottery "seconds" along side Audrey's new tablecloths. Surprisingly the Poole pottery was cheaper than acquiring new crockery from Ministry suppliers. These, together with other small changes, were to the delight of our regular volunteers and helped to maintain a good recruitment through their recommendations to family and friends on their return home.

During Mrs Andrews' stay the trials became more involved, making it difficult for her to carry out the duties required. The result being that on her retirement two nursing officers were employed to carry out these duties.

Mrs A. Dalton who lived on site with her husband, daughter and son, and Miss J. Dunning who lived locally were sadly to be the last of Harvard's "gracious" matrons. Each one had her own ideas, which sometimes presented me with a challenge, but equally each one is remembered for her contribution to Harvard.

Kitchen And Catering

Reading the many verses the volunteers have written, it shows they looked forward to the porter's food trolley and its contents, and were, on the whole satisfied with what they had. A weekly menu sheet was available, volunteers could if they wished have one, but most declined, preferring the element of surprise.

Matron, whilst on her morning round, took note of any likes and dislikes. The general comment was that perhaps the meals were too large, although the young teenage students had healthy appetites and often requested bigger helpings!

Each volunteer flat had its kitchen/diner equipped with crockery, cutlery, condiments, electric kettle, hot plate, fridge, milk saucepan, toaster and bread bin. Each flat had a sink unit with hot and cold running water. Washing up liquid, cloths, mops, bucket and general household cleaning materials were also supplied.

On the Monday morning prior to the trial starting on the Tuesday the kitchen was stocked with coffee, tea, sugar, breakfast cereal, jam, marmalade, tomato and brown sauce, eggs, milk, butter, bread and tins of soup. As already mentioned the trial started after lunch on the Tuesday with the majority of the volunteers arriving during the morning. For those with long distances to travel, making a morning arrival difficult, arrangements were made for them to take up residence during the previous evening, with a cold supper being provided. Often, however, these volunteers would tour Salisbury and have a meal in town.

On intake day all volunteers had lunch in the dining room with members of staff which enabled everyone to become acquainted. These were very friendly affairs and after coffee had been served the introductory talk was given by the Medical Superintendent, Matron and the Executive Officer.

These talks were designed to give the volunteers an outline of

51

the experiment, isolation procedures, games and sports facilities, the best country walks and how to make the best use of their flat facilities, especially their kitchen and meals. Volunteers who had been many times were well acquainted with these talks and would often tell us if we had missed anything out!

Following the talk volunteers were taken to the local hospital unit for chest X-Ray's, this was a safeguard against chest infection both for the volunteers and the Harvard establishment.

All meals from there on were delivered to the volunteers' flats in thermos containers for hot food, the cold sweets, cakes, fruits etc., in heavy plastic boxes. Each thermos container housed four separate dishes, one for meat, the second, third and fourth for vegetables and hot sweets. Two food containers, suitably marked, plus the four inner dishes served each flat. The empties were collected on delivery of the next meal. Each flat had its

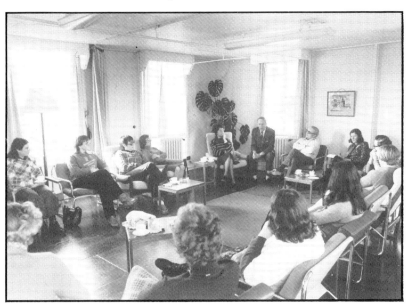

Dr Craig (under the far window) explaining the coming trial after the Intake Day lunch.

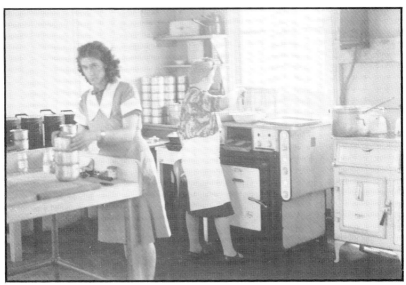

Above and below: Preparing the meals for volunteers.

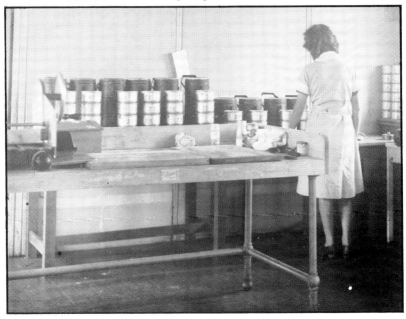

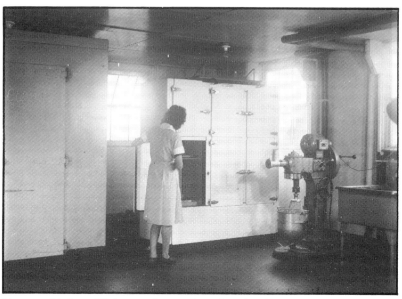

Above and below: Kitchen equipment from America. The cold room/large fridge was still in use in 1990.

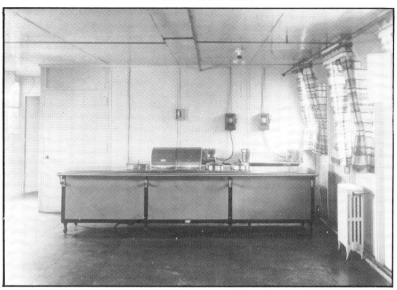

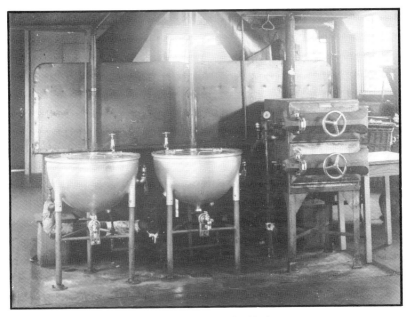

Above and below: in the kitchen.

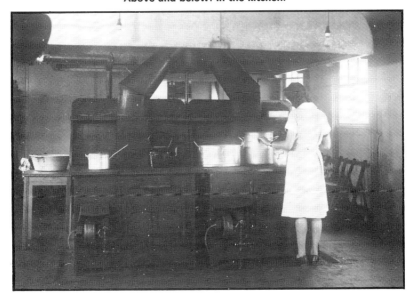

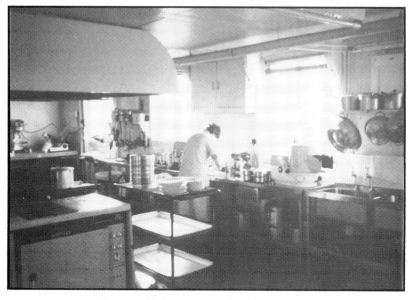

Above and below: The modernised kitchens.

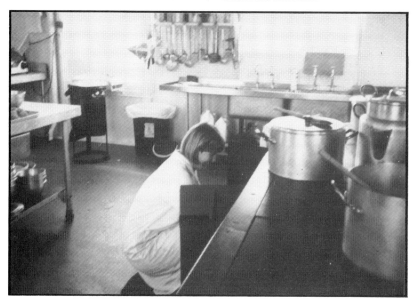

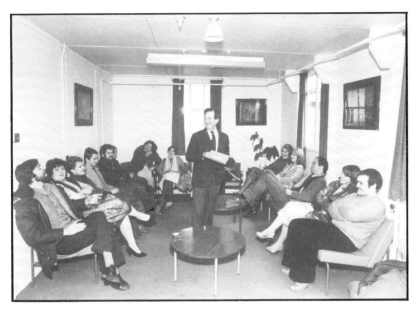

Virologist Dr A. S. Beare sharing a joke with volunteers during a pre-trial briefing.

own containers as part of the isolation procedure. The porter delivering the meal would give one ring on the door bell, the "inmate" waiting until his departure before going to the door thus preventing close contact. (When matron, doctors and laboratory staff visited the flats they rang twice on the door bell and walked in, suitably masked and gowned.)

The catering staff were on duty throughout the ten day trials with the exception of Saturday and Sunday evening meals. On those days in the summer a salad was provided and in the winter a pre-cooked meal was taken in an electrically heated pan, which they could re-heat themselves. Three cooked meals a day were available if required, however many volunteers had just toast and cereal for breakfast, or perhaps a boiled egg using their own kitchen facilities. Throughout the Harvard lifespan the standard of catering was very good with few complaints, which were usually simple to solve.

Three chefs served the Unit. The first, Mr Cameron Clarke,

57

who in 1953 transferred to the Administration. Miss Gwen Ray took his place, being promoted from assistant cook. Miss Ray lived on the Unit with her mother who gave piano lessons to the residents' children. Miss Ray retired in 1974 after 22 years of dedicated service.

Mr Steve Hall followed Miss Ray, transferring from Salisbury General Infirmary and remaining in service until the Unit's closure. Steve and Miss Ray, like so many of the Unit's staff, were always willing to help if needed with work other than their own. One particular incident comes to mind, when they delivered the volunteers' meals by sledge when the Unit became snowbound during the winters of 1947 and 1963.

Until 1960 resident families had their meals cooked by the Harvard kitchen, for it was considered that electric ovens were too big a fire risk because of the wooden construction of the buildings. Mid-day and evening meals were collected from the kitchen at the appropriate time, payment for this service being made to the office on a weekly/monthly basis. The cooking of meals for resident staff was a novelty at first, eventually causing many problems due primarily to the time-table and occasionally the menu.

In many establishments of institutional catering one could tell the day of the week by the menu. This was discouraged at Harvard. It was, however, an embarrassment to hear a volunteer comment that the menus were a repeat of their last visit, and, of course, it was impossible to please everyone.

Many of the cooking untensils sent over with the hospital from America were still in use and in good working order at the Unit's closure, including tables, walk-in cold room and 16ft long hot servery. After 43 years continuous use it says a great deal for the standard of workmanship.

Volunteers, Why They Came And Their Comments

Following the initial inquiry a potential volunteer received an application form, list of trial dates together with letters giving a detailed account of the Unit, conditions for volunteers, facilities at the Unit, research procedures, experimental methods and the important isolation procedures.

There are many varied reasons why people volunteered. Some, but few, came for purely scientific reasons, others came "to get away from it all" and after the first visit when they experienced such peace, tranquillity and a homely atmosphere many returned time and time again. It's coming the first time which is commendable, I would think in the lifetime of Harvard hundreds of would be volunteers have decided to come, then been dissuaded by relatives and friends. Many said they saw it advertised years before they came, and then were reminded when reading a magazine in a doctor's or dentist's waiting room or under the dryer at the hairdresser. Nurses found it helpful to unwind. We had many visits from a husband and wife, proprietors of a busy seaside resort fish and chip establishment. Students came prepared with books to do a lot of studying during their stay, but there was no doubt that the delights of the countryside as well as the joys of doing nothing often conspired to defeat these good intentions.

During the post-war period queueing for rations at shops was common to everyone but not those at Harvard as this was all done for them. Letters of appreciation came from a large number of volunteers with such comments as "I thought I would give it a try and I have been five times since." "I first heard of Harvard at school from my head teacher and became a volunteer on reaching the age of 18, liking it but not coming again for 10 years after getting married and having children."

One housewife said sadly that after donating her still born baby to medical science she thought she should do more to help research and came to Harvard. Another, out of work, saw a notice in the Job Centre asking for volunteers and enrolled. "I was very depressed after a divorce and coming to Harvard helped me a lot," commented another. Many came after a death in the family, loss of a job, moving away from lifetime friends and family, loss of husband or wife and for many other personal reasons.

There were far more happier reasons such as "We had just got married and could not afford an expensive honeymoon," or "We have bought a house with a large mortgage and this is a cheap holiday for us. It is ideal countryside to study the flora and fauna, I came to paint landscapes, or study local churches." Volunteers were allowed in the village churches without breaking isolation rules — looking into the church first — but most village churches were empty during weekdays. Another couple wrote "We met at Harvard and after marrying have been coming every year since, but not next year as we are starting a family." Some, after the end of the trial, went on for a week's holiday in a south coast resort, coming from a northern town they had their train fares or car expenses paid to and from their home town to Salisbury by the Unit. Many did various jobs that they could not normally do at home, such as dressmaking, or learning to dressmake, knitting intricate patterns needing complete concentration, athletes practising for sprint events and one or two during the summer months carried out maintenance on their cars. "There is so much room at Harvard so I brought my sewing machine to make curtains for the house," said one lady, others brought their knitting machines and one good lady her spinning wheel.

A taxi driver who was accepted as a volunteer and not informing his wife left a note for her saying "Gone to Harvard, back in 10 days!"

A wayfarer called at the office asking if he could take part in the trials. Fortunately it was intake day and Dr Craig, the Medical Superintendent said "Yes." After a change of clothing, a rest and good food he was a successful volunteer and came again.

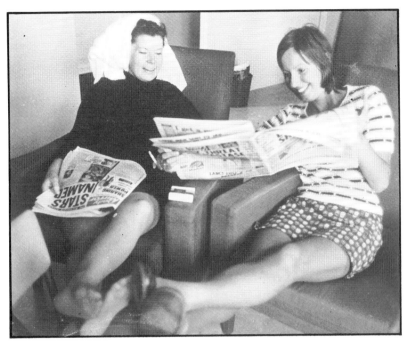

Above: A couple of volunteers enjoying the daily papers.

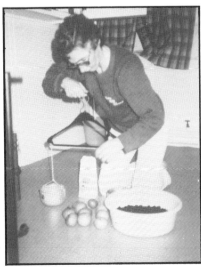

Right: Using coat-hanger scales to weigh the ingredients for blackberry and apple jam.

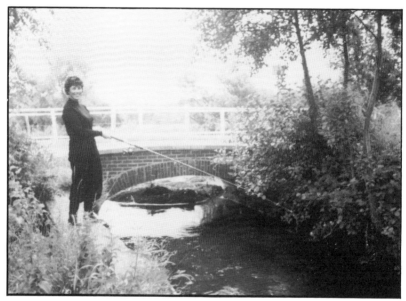

A volunteer fishing at Britford, near Salisbury.

The following is a typical example of why people came. The girl was an impoverished student nurse who could not afford a holiday but needed one and by coming to Harvard might in some way be benefiting others. "Although the Unit never managed but a sniffle in me, the sheer bliss of not being available at the end of a phone, the peace and quiet at Harvard has always been a valve to my otherwise busy life," writes another satisfied volunteer.

"In my nine visits, at 'pocket money time' I always felt I should be paying for the complete relaxation one feels at the end of the trial" writes Jennifer Holloway from Tipton. "Without the concentrated time available to me at Harvard for several years I would not now have my Open University B.A. degree." Jennifer went on to say that on one trial when sharing with two undergraduates, one who had brought her computer, the other studying for her S.R.N. finals, "We discussed for hours examinations and techniques on courses we had taken, which was very enlightening to me and helped me in my further studies." In conclusion Jennifer said that on every occasion she got on well with her flat mates.

Talking to other volunteers they were also pleased with their acquaintances, commending the Harvard team for successfully pairing off perfect strangers. One student nurse mentions the country walks, her favourite being to Longford Castle via the Heronry, always a source of fascination. Never a keen sportswoman, but because of the relaxed atmosphere at Harvard, she always sampled badminton, padder tennis, snooker, table tennis, golf etc. She said "It may seem that the purpose of the trials from a volunteer's point of view may have been unimportant, but this was not true at all. The trials themselves were a constant source of interest. All the staff have been unfailingly kind and helpful and this undoubtedly has

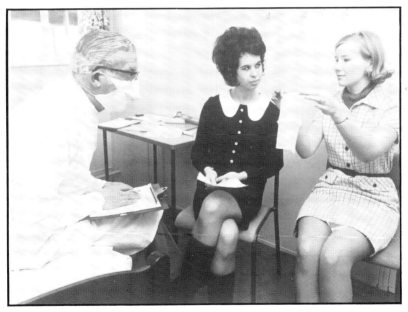

Handkerchief inspection by Dr Hall during his morning round (photograph courtesy of Fox Photos Ltd).

influenced volunteers to return many times over. Like the Royal Family, it must be difficult to always show interest and be friendly to a changing succession of people."

Joy Haslem from Derby a volunteer at no less than 16 trials, explained that her first visit with a cousin was one of adventure, excitement and apprehension which mounted as the train drew into Salisbury Station. "Being assured and put at ease by the driver collecting us from the station, we realized that there was no turning back now. Things we had discussed for weeks, i.e. food, beds, living accommodation, Harvard staff, these worries soon disappeared with the 10 days passing all too quickly. The sun shone continuously and we got fatter and browner by the day. The days were spent playing games, walking, reading and writing to friends and relatives who had tried to stop us coming, but thank goodness they failed. We assured them of our continuing good health. As we packed our cases to leave, two things were certain, we had loved it and would certainly be

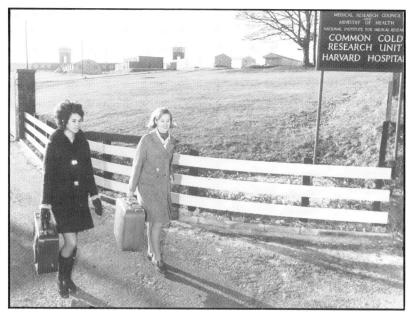

Two volunteers leave for home (photograph courtesy of Fox Photos Ltd).

back! Although over the next 16 years the apprehension of that first visit disappeared, the excitement never left us. It always reached fever pitch on changing trains at Bristol Temple Meads Station where the accent of the station announcer made me feel I was 'almost home'.''

Our two volunteers go on to mention some of the staff. First, Audrey Rogers who shopped for them, as ever attentive to their needs. Dennis, the groundsman, meticulously tending his flower beds and grass. Steve Hall — chef — responsible for their disappearing waistlines. Angela Simms, from the office paying out the "pocket money". Lastly, Kathy Brown chief laboratory technician, coming to the volunteers with her pipettes, viruses and saline lotions.

They mention the disappointment of leaving Harvard at the end of the trial and returning to the "outside world" where unmasked and ungowned "Aliens" come closer than 30 ft! A short rehabilitation course to prepare them for the outside world would have been ideal. Lastly, finding a substitute for my annual Harvard holiday is going to be impossible. We would willingly volunteer our services for any other research projects, the Chocolate Research Council perhaps!

I've heard volunteers describe Harvard as Typically British, so few rules, with no signs to indicate isolation areas. This information was given at the briefing on arrival. Over the years and with successive administrations everything had been done to keep things as relaxed and informal as possible. No one demands to see your birth certificate, people are taken that "my word is my bond" and the trials are carried out in a relaxed atmosphere.

People, of course, had their favourite flats, as one mentioned "I'm a 6B man," another a 3A and so on. One volunteer complained his toilet was blocked, after moving him into another flat, which turned out to be his favourite, on investigation the problem we found he had stuffed his loo with wild watercress from the nearby stream! 1A it seems is down as the "Nosey flat," so much can be seen from there.

Another volunteer stated "I found an advertisement for Harvard in a book called *Alternative Holidays*" another "I came to

Harvard to write my annual Christmas letters sent to relatives. To each I write the happenings of that period and in December I complete it into one long letter sending perhaps a dozen of them to relations, all this being done at Harvard." A husband and wife said they saw the need for volunteers in *The Lady* magazine — "It tickled our sense of humour so we gave it a go. We arrived for the first time on our motor bikes, stopped at the entrance, it all looked forbidding, those two black water towers and Nissen huts, we nearly turned back, but of course we were shown our accommodation and seeing the fantastic views from our sitting room window we fell in love with the place."

"We used to bring stacks and stacks of paperwork to do, but now we do nothing, just soak in the atmosphere."

"I was stationed on Salisbury Plain in the A.T.S. and used to pass Harvard going home on the bus and thought I must go there one day — and here I am six years later on my fourth visit."

In a similar situation, when asking a 19 year old student if she had been before, "Oh, I'm the third generation" she replied, "My grandparents came in the early 50s, followed by my parents many years later and now me. My grandparents asked me to discover if Tom was still there — are you him?" "Yes" I replied, deflated at realizing my age.

"Coming to Harvard fulfilled a New Year's resolution," replied one satisfied volunteer, wishing she had come before. Many people passed the Unit on their way to West Country holidays, one could not miss the large sign at the entrance which read "Medical Research Council Common Cold Unit." Few were curious and made enquiries resulting in their becoming volunteers at a later date.

One such student remembers during a trial taking part in a strange party. Intimate it was not. "We sat in a ring at 30ft intervals, conversed in decibels and were served cake by gentlemen masked and gowned in white. We could easily have been taken for a gathering of Druids, after all we were not far from Stonehenge. We then took part in musical chairs and under these conditions it took on an Alice In Wonderland concept, a combination of the Mad Hatter's Tea party and the confusion of the games in the Queen of Hearts' Garden as we ran from deck chair to deck chair. I must have been mad taking part in such a weird game, or even coming here at all after having spent a small fortune on thermal underwear and vitamins this winter to ward off a cold, now I am asking to catch one!"

An employee of the manufacturers Ravenhead Glass came on a trial and as we normally did after the lunch on the last day handed out leaflets to be put on works notice boards etc. This lad took quite a number, saying he would put them in the glassware packing cases. He was true to his word, for sometime later two hotel employees from Bristol arrived having learnt of Harvard after unpacking a carton of glasses and finding our leaflets.

Another volunteer, who lived in Salisbury, has been coming for six years and although a native of the area, she explained

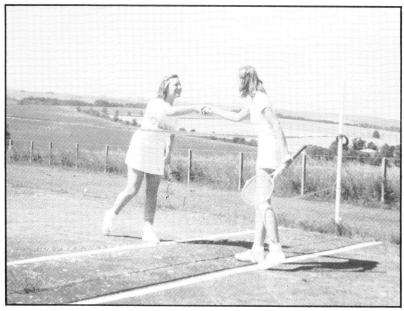

Volunteers meet for a friendly game of tennis. The Wiltshire Downs are in the background.

67

"One sees the locality from an entirely new angle, the view is panoramic when looking down on Odstock," the village in which she was born.

Mrs Margaret Goodall attended her first trial as a volunteer in 1972, but by 1983 she had made 15 visits, co-opted 22 members of her family, neighbours and workmates, many of whom also made annual visits. They included: mum, sisters, brothers, uncles, nephews and in-laws.

For several years ten came down from Scotland to Harvard by hired mini-bus, booking five of the volunteer flats at a time. They were a friendly crowd and I was proud to have been accepted as one of the "family." In 1982 they came to Harvard especially early to present me with a retirement present and card from all the family of which I am justly proud.

"My sister encouraged me to come and seeing me off on the bus, with one foot on its step she told me of the nasal washings. I immediately panicked and tried to get off but was pushed on by the passenger behind who shouted "Come on lady, we haven't got all day," so here I am on my 12th visit.

The grandstand on Salisbury Racecourse can be clearly seen from Harvard and on race days volunteers who liked the odd flutter would have a bet and this was done for them by Audrey as part of her daily volunteer shopping expeditions. A lady volunteer studying form saw a runner named "Duck 'n Dive." "I must do this, as I've been ducking and diving to avoid breaking isolation ever since I've been here." Sure enough a clear winner at 10—1, so the lady went home happy with a few extra pounds.

Lots of volunteers are saying they had a feeling of pride to assist and be actively involved in such important scientific work, there was the aspect of feeling "useful" and the desire to help others which is in most people's nature. We learned to live with people we would not normally choose to meet. The difference in dialect, humour and the character building aspect of communal type life.

Besides the high praise for the Harvard staff, volunteers say they will have lasting memories. Perhaps, of late sunny afternoons curled in the armchair, reading and filling in the shopping forms, looking through the library list deciding which books to request. The snooker or table tennis which was played in a World War II Nissen hut, full with the ghosts of servicemen, the creaking of the beds, the sound of footsteps on the wooden walkways. The bang of the box lid as the porter puts in the enormous food flask with the latest meal, the angry ring that is managed to be produced if we had not put in the empty flask.

"My first walk of each trial is down through those lovely villages, or sitting on the verandah like an 'Old Colonial' watching the sunset, looking through the scrap books, the friendliness and humour of the place, finally the ability to be perfectly still and let go of life, the strength and healing power of absolute silence. Every year going home refreshed, each winter getting out my Salisbury South Ordnance Survey Map and planning my walks for the next summer's Harvard visit."
Some Harvard staff recommended their friends and relatives to take part in the trials. Sir Christopher Andrewes' son, John, came on three occasions, he met a girl who took part in the first trial. They remained friends over the years and he is now Godfather to one of her daughters. During his days at Cambridge University John became a recruiting agent for Harvard.

My younger son also took part on two occasions, the second time being the final trial No. 1006 from 18–27 July 1989. A sentimental experience for him since he was born on the Unit. During coffee after the intake day lunch a young lady asked him if he had been to Harvard before? "Yes, I was born here." Thinking he was being sarcastic she left her seat beside him, and sitting by another volunteer said "That chap thinks I'm an idiot!"

"Harvard became a family 'must' " explains one lad after his fourth visit, "My parents came in the 60s, my older brother in the 70s, and now me in the 80s. It was natural for me to come to Harvard."

Three ladies came regularly about the same time each year and made jam. They were nicknamed "the jam makers" and gave samples of their jam to the staff.

We received a letter telling us how the writer and his friend

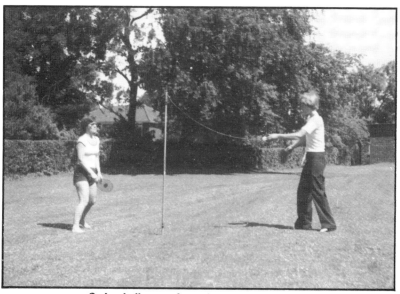

Swing-ball was a favourite with volunteers.

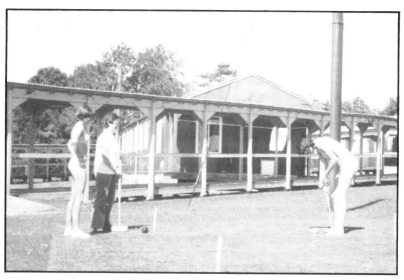

Croquet, another favourite pastime, needed concentration.

had attended a trial, met two ladies and subsequently had a double wedding, followed by a honeymoon at the Unit.

One could continue recording comments of volunteers. This one I particularly like; it involves a 19 year old lad, who since the age of 10 had journeyed alone by train from his London home each summer to visit his aunt in Basingstoke for two weeks' holiday. On this occasion he found himself at Harvard taking part in a common cold trial. At Waterloo Station he purchased his return ticket to Basingstoke and settled in the carriage as he had done for the past 10 years. A lady entered the compartment and seating herself opposite him began telling him of her annual trip to Harvard and how good it was. Before reaching Basingstoke, which was approximately half way from Waterloo to Salisbury, the lady had persuaded him to continue on to Harvard, which he did paying the excess fare on arrival at Salisbury. Luckily he was medically fit and also there was room on the trial for him. And so another volunteer was duly accommodated. Naturally his family were somewhat surprised when he telephoned explaining his sudden change of plan.

Ninety-nine per cent of volunteers coming to the Unit enjoyed their stay, but of course there were the inevitable problems. A handful were mis-matched, and had to be re-flatted, I cannot remember anyone having "fisty-cuffs," but I recall that one volunteer broke his ankle jumping from a high walkway returning home.

There was an occasion in the early days when a volunteer turned burglar when end of Trial parties were held in the dining room. He, of course, did not attend but waited until the party was in full swing and then made the rounds of the volunteers' flats and secured a profitable haul. In one flat he confronted a girl who had not attended the party, having a sore throat, the burglar made the excuse he had been sent to correct an electrical fault, the girl was suspicious and helped us to give the Police his details. He was caught on a subsequent occasion and asked for the Harvard burglaries to be taken into consideration.

Breaking the isolation procedure and being sent home in disgrace was always a sad event, both for the volunteer and staff. Depending on the circumstances the offending volunteer was "black listed" and could not attend again, some were caught in town shopping, others in the "local" having a drink.

The Medical Superintendent, living on site at the time went to the Rose and Crown one evening. On the way back he passed a volunteer going to the Rose and Crown. The Medical Superintendent told him he would see him in the morning, but the volunteer left before morning. Three volunteers went to the Yew Tree for a drink at lunchtime, unfortunately for them, two members of staff were there, celebrating a birthday.

Members of the opposite sexes were caught associating together, although, this like all breaking of isolation procedures was rare. I recall an incident when lads flatted at one end and girls at the opposite end of the same building cohabited. The lads had crawled through the ceiling panels and then along the roof space to drop into the girls, flat next door. One couple having been told they could go for walks together providing they kept a distance of 30 feet, used a piece of string that length as a guide, but the string (so we were told) became entangled around a tree bringing the couple "face to face!"

The number of volunteers who broke isolation were few. During the introductory talk they were warned that if isolation was broken they would be sent home without 'pocket money,' also they would not be allowed to come again, they were then given the opportunity to go home if they felt the rules of isolation would be too stringent for them. I do not remember anyone leaving on intake day.

One volunteer during a walk used his penknife to cut a stick and succeeded in cutting himself as well. Bleeding profusely, but still aware of the 30 feet limit he attracted the attention of a car driver and asked her to ring the Unit but insisted that she didn't come near him. On the phone the poor girl seemed rather bewildered by his attitude! One of our nursing sisters and the driver went to collect the volunteer and took him to hospital to have his wound, a cut tendon, stitched. Unfortunately, isolation was breeched, although the volunteer had tried so hard to maintain isolation.

One young lady asked to go home giving the reason of falling desperately in love with a married man attending the trial with

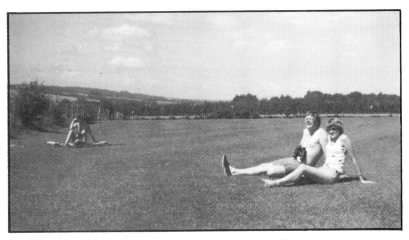

Volunteers relaxing in the sun (1978).

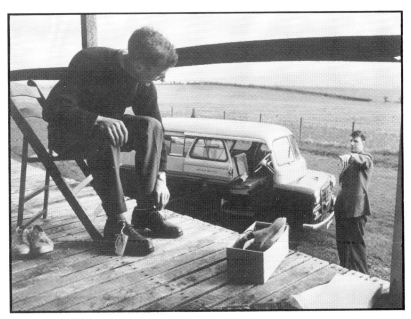

A volunteer tries on a pair of walking shoes, obtained on approval — all part of the "Harvard service".

73

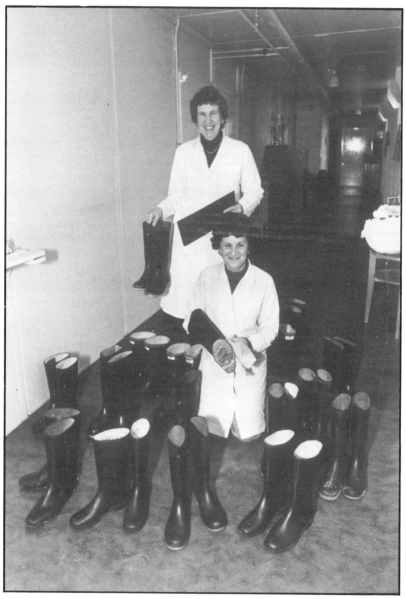

Audrey Rogers and Pearl Safe preparing "wellies" for a trial.

his wife. She had apparently sat next to him at the intake day lunch. Going home, she said, was the only solution in getting him out of her mind.

Another chap thinking he had been unfairly treated went home because we could not supply a Communist newspaper on the day of issue.

Few would be volunteers had not been truthful in answering the questions on their application forms. On their arrival it was obvious that they would not make good volunteers as they were much too old or unfortunately socially unacceptable. They were suitably reimbursed for any inconvenience and then were encouraged to return home. On one occasion the man in question had no home to which he could return. I met him several times afterwards in Salisbury and eventually he found work in the town.

On an application form a volunteer put "teacher" as her occupation. During conversations with the nursing sisters she said she used to teach but, on the Sunday of the trial she received a phone call and left the unit. Apparently she was a journalist and left because she was needed for another assignment.

Another volunteer on her first visit put the year of her birth as 1936. Two visits later it was changed to 1937, then next time it was back to 1936. Each visit therafter her year of birth went up by one. She never reached the 50 age limit, but remained at 49 according to her form.

During his term in office Dr Bynoe accepted two totally blind men as volunteers, they came with high recommendations from the Association for the Blind. After being enrolled and shown the details of their accommodation and the adjacent outside area was explained they became excellent volunteers causing no problems whatsoever. Their flat was left clean and in good order at the end of the trial.

A young lady confined to a wheelchair was also accepted. She was housed in an accessible flat, but it was necessary to build a small concrete ramp for easy access. She caused quite a problem at the end of the trial when her parents came to take her home by locking herself in the bedroom, persuasion had no effect, neither did the master key. A forced entry had to be made and the poor lady left the Unit in floods of tears.

It was necessary for the administration to continually use all methods available to ensure a good supply of applicants to become volunteers, giving the Medical Superintendent as large a number as possible from which to make his selection and thereby reduce the likelihood of a possible unwise choice.

Cures And Curios

It was always interesting to listen to the laboratory staff talking about the research currently in progress during the coffee/meal breaks and also how the volunteers were being used during each trial. The elation when experiments were proceeding well and the need for that extra cup of Harvard's strong coffee when results were not so good.

Not being a scientist I would not attempt to comment on the complex work carried out at Harvard, this will no doubt be done by Dr Tyrrell in a more comprehensive book on the Unit's work.

Hundreds of suggestions were sent in over the years by members of the public for the prevention or cure of the common cold. Some obviously used by our grandmothers were debatable, others funny, even mind boggling, others most definitely macabre. The following are all a mixture of suggested cures and prevention in no specific order:—

Gargle with malt vinegar swallowing about two teaspoons night and morning.

Make a preserve of dried prunes, fresh pears and lemons and eat on bread for breakfast and at teatime.

From Australia came the request for a cure by September 1946, some task since the Unit's first Trial was in July of that year.

The preclusion of light — this is difficult to assess whether prevention or cure, it sounds more like a punishment.

An electrical massage.

Do not wear socks or stockings.

This gem was from a Parisian who suggested the inhalation of small amounts of First World War gases.

Don't read or listen to the weather forecast — very sensible — would be prevention or cure of many maladies.

We were informed that the Common Cold was not caused by a virus but from eating indigestible food.

When feeling a cold use nose rings — not the metal type, but pieces of cotton wool placed in each nostril — handy for decorating the Christmas tree by sneezing!

Cut the feet off socks or stockings and wear only leather boots or shoes, this also cures chilblains.

Inhale smelling salts four times a day.

A person wrote to tell us that he could produce a cold at anytime by inhaling the fumes from a frying pan. He omitted to tell us what he was frying, or how often he did it. When needing time off work no doubt.

Everyone should be his own doctor says another. Take and do what he thinks for a cure. I suppose many of us do that. For instance some prefer one brand of whisky to another as an excuse for a cure.

Inhale fumes from photographic developer.

Sensible I thought is the suggestion to gargle salt saline solution.

Strips of gauze or cotton wool placed between the toes.

We'll furnish you with a cure if you forward the sum of ten guineas — there's enterprise and confidence for you!

Drink Horlicks before going to bed.

This one should cure the cold with a BANG! The suggestion washing your mouth out with petrol!

Certain types of slimming pills are a good cure.

This next one I follow myself, taking Cod Liver Oil capsules night and morning.

Eat plenty of Marmite and raw beef steaks.

Shake the head from side to side twice a day says a young lady — leaving the cold somewhere in the middle no doubt.

Mix olive oil with oil of cloves and place 10 drops in each ear twice daily.

Breathe sea water into the nostrils — seems a good excuse to have a coastal holiday during a cold or to live by the sea as a prevention.

Sit under a photographic arc light for one hour each day.

Wash nostrils out with soapy water each morning.

Convert the smallest room in the house into a hot chamber and sit in it for one hour each day.

Take a turkish bath each day.

The suggestion to prevent a cold by not living in Manchester could cause a mass exodus from that fine city.

Make wax tablets mixed with natural oils and hang one in each room of the house — giving five year olds something to do on a rainy day I suppose.

Keep away from spiders' webs.

Give up smoking — a very sensible idea.

The idea of not to blow your nose during a cold as a cure gives Tupperware scope to design an under nostril drip tray!

To gargle a mixture of salt and bicarbonate of soda doesn't seem too bad.

Inhale a mild form of insecticide when fumigating the greenhouse.

The man who suggested that a good prevention is to breathe in female body odour doesn't state how often or how first to catch your female.

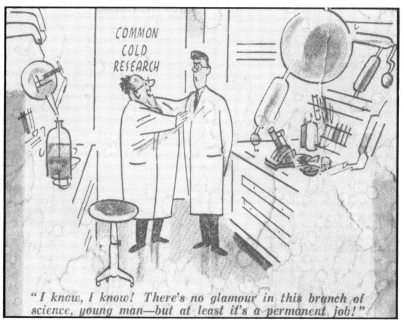

Cartoon titled "What a life!"

Don't drink tea, coffee or mineral waters.

Take lots of Vitamin B and eat wholemeal bread.

The following four recommendations must have collaborated for a cure. Inhale fumes from: Bread Yeast, Charcoals, DDT, Welding Copper.

This last one was suggested by an acquaintance of mine who did some copper welding at the Harvard Laboratories in 1948 and has never since suffered a cold.

Wear a flannel undergarment impregnated with sodium sulphate.

Don't wash your hair during a cold.

Take a spoonful of glycerine with a dash of lime juice.

I wonder how the chap came up with the following — that honeymoon couples don't get colds because of the warmth of their love.

The recommendation to massage into the hair a mixture of ammonia, turpentine and spirits of Camphor, inhaling from the hands before washing suggests he didn't want any friends.

Use strong soap in the bath.

Don't eat any kind of meat.

So we continue to the lady who suggested the best cure was to go to bed for an hour after arriving home from work.

Stand in the cold for five minutes following a bath.

Place a nutmeg in each sock.

Do not drink alcohol in any form or smoke and remain unmarried, which is in total contrast to the following words of wisdom!

Drink one large gin, two large rums followed by a meal of grass cutlets wash down with four pints of strong ale. Recommending that the grass in the cutlets be of good quality.

A more gentle suggestion is to sit each evening with a cat on your lap.

Take a shower night and morning.

Avoid bread and potatoes.

Use an infra red lamp.

Don't have freshly killed pork in the house.

Drink TCP mixed with water.

Take half a calcium sulphate tablet twice daily.

Eat a large onion boiled in milk.

Inhale smoke from the burning autumn leaves of a bonfire.

Become a Blood Donor.

Use garlic whenever possible.

The last group of remedies seems harmless to try.
We finish the recommended cures and prevention with more venturous or hazardous suggestions, namely:—

To kiss a mule on the nose.

Bee keeping prevents colds.

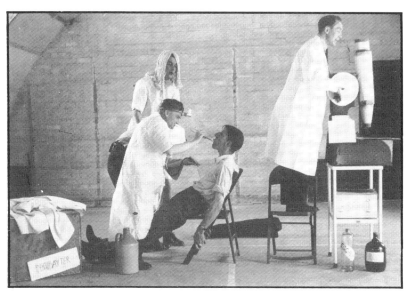

A spoof depiction of "a virologist in serious study".

Put stale bread in old worn socks and hang round one's neck.

Chop up leaves from wild horehound, mix with honey and eat slowly.

Take a spoonful of goose grease before going to bed.

Smear nostrils with rheumatic balm.

Sniff a pinch of bicarbonate of soda every hour.

Mix in mice when making a casserole.

Cobwebs eaten between two slices of apple.

Lastly, to wear slippers until very old with toes sticking out, then place in bed before going to sleep.

These are only a small sample of preventions and cures contained in letters sent to the Unit during its existence, none are made up by me. It is left to the reader to decide which are a figment of the imagination, fiction, ludicrous, worth trying, ethical, psychological or what grandmother always did.

Some letters were a genuine plea for help from people who had continuous colds wishing the Unit success in finding a cure and passing it on to them as soon as possible.

> Dramatic medical advance to unfold
> But here sit I with my common cold

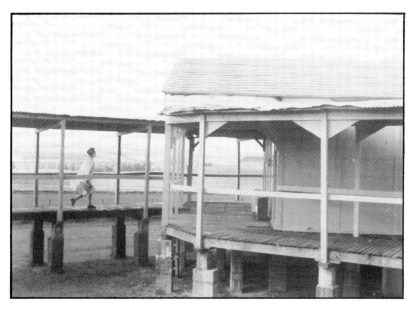

Matron M. Turnbull, facing the elements, on her morning round of visiting volunteers.

From The Scrapbook

The following pieces of prose and poetry are taken from a scrapbook kept at the Unit by volunteers.

"Mary's story"

Long walks in wellies and a headscarf. Too much to eat and all of it fattening. A simple routine of living from meal to meal and matron's visit, an exercise bicycle, grey mistiness over the countryside and a flurry of paws on the other side of the hedge.

A duck startled off her nest by the roadside because I had stepped aside for a lorry, the lorry driver's face and the shouted conversation about ducks.

The man in the red anorak sitting in his back garden smoking a cigarette. I had taken him for a piece of equipment and was amazed when he said "Good morning."

A line of broken, dishevelled caravans in the lane, the children and barking dogs, a zinc bath of water over a wood fire and an old roller mangle standing by for the washing.

Pretty cottages in the village, neatly done up by Solicitors or architects. The village church with its *Hymns Ancient And Modern* and the *Book Of Common Prayer* and the familiar smell of stone and wood and faintly rotting kneelers.

Wooden slatted walk-ways that go round the chalets, covered with corrugated roofs and pale green beams. The noise people make when they walk along them from hut to hut. Faces that look out to see who is on the walk-way because a new passer by is an experience.

Matron's red watering can beside her door and the eyes that must, by now, over her white mask, have learnt to convey more than eyes normally do.

The privacy of a room which is mine, a bed with heavy, white cotton sheets that smell delicious, the freedom of knowing I may put on the light to read in the middle of the night.

The facility to lie perfectly still and let go of life. The strength and healing power of absolute silence.

I love it here.

Mary Langley
March 1980

The Housewives
We are three housewives pure and simple,
None of us pure and all of us simple!
We set up house in Flat 3A,
For ten whole days we had come to stay.

Oh! Come to Harvard and catch a cold!
It's not very likely, that's what we were told.
No menus to dream up every day.
We'd have free time to go and play!

The Aussie film crew made Lesley's eyes gleam,
They really were a fabulous team.
Her wish for a chat nearly drew a blank,
Last seen she was shinning up the water tank!

Jill's gaze fell in another direction,
To her the young porter was perfection.
Imagine her dismay to see him with a wife (?)
She nearly resorted to crime — with a knife!

To Marilyn fell the most difficult task,
For padlocks and chains on her list she did ask.
She pleaded with Matron to keep them in check,
They plotted at midnight to wring her darned neck!

We're on our way now, after many a spree,
The cold germs and food were abundant — and free!
The staff were so friendly, but now need a rest.
"We'll be back", the three threatened, but was it in jest?

Jill, Lesley, Marilyn
Trial 839
May 1982

Who Cares?
I throw off me girdle — me bra off too,
Me Stiletto's I kicks off with glee
No make up plastered on me face
Yes Darlin *this* is me

A sniff and a sneeze in warm summer breeze
Rolled over me shorts is me belly.
I eats like a horse, then sits down and smokes
Feet up and on with the telly.

Who cares what I looks like, or cares what I does?
There's nobody cares more than me.
But here I will lazy, for next ten days
Oh, Lordy! It's great to feel free.

Me Darlin has never seen me like this
And stares at me in right dismay
Can I have married this wretched slag?
No he smiles "I like you this way"

Babs Wilde
Trial 823 — 1981

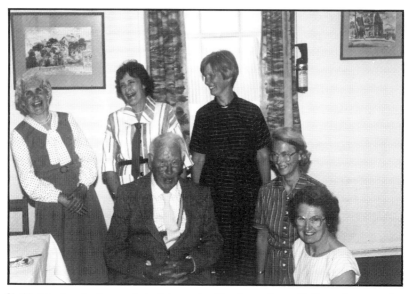

Sir Christopher Andrewes, in jovial mood, with a bevy of past Ph.D. students, on the occasion of his 90th birthday.

A Volunteer's Eye View
Some wonderous stories I could tell,
'Bout Harvard C.C.U.,
About volunteers who caught a cold
And those who got the 'flu.

We see the porter passing by,
With wine and cans of beer,
(Not for us, we're staying dry) HA HA!
Some-one is full of cheer.

The food we get is wonderful,
We didn't ask for more,
But alas, there's something wrong,
I can't get through the door.

The doctor comes round every morn,
With Matron in his wake,
"Now, any symptoms?" he enquires,
"The truth, and please don't fake".

Now two rings on the doorbell,
Who's that? Oh golly gosh,
I'm naked in the shower and
It's time for a nasal wash.

"Head back" says Helen gaily,
As she squirts stuff up my nose,
She counts each drop back in the dish,
As down my nose it flows.

Our shopping, done by Audrey,
The stuff for us she brought,
I know that when we settle up,
My balance will be naught.

My flatmate Ruth's gone walking,
With wellies on her feet,
I'm sitting with my feet up,
Oh what a lovely treat.

I ring the office daily,
"More books! More books!" I plead,
I don't come here to catch a cold,
I only come to read".

But now the trials' nearly done,
Our books we must return,
A last meal in the dining room,
"No sweet" I must be firm.

And now the time has come to leave,
A last glimpse through the gate,
But I'll be back again, don't fear,

Till next year I must wait.

Gill Tanner
Trial 834
February 1982

Volunteers Last Day

It was a raging, noisesome, roaring day
With a wounded wind torn and tearing
about the confines of a lowered sky
When you were whisked away into
tumultuous life, into the hurly burl of everyday
to face the storms of normal, real.
Rested in the brief calm of holiday
Towards the viscious nightmare of unsheltered bright.
Toward the next shelter from the storm
To join the ones you love
Leaving company and shared times
Touched trees, calling birds, walked fields
and mainly people.
We wend our ways apart, to later
Unwind memory in differing isolations.
Take love and comfort with you
Always.

Eileen Glynn
Trial 829
November 1981

The Ebble Valley Study

In 1948 fieldwork was carried out by the Harvard scientists to collect information on the spread of colds through the community. There is a string of villages and hamlets stretching for about 12 miles along the Chalk Valley through which runs the Ebble, a tributary of the beautiful River Avon. The valley was ideal for the study of the transmitting of colds as it was but a short distance from the Common Cold Research Unit.

The first of the 15 villages is Bodenham lying two miles south of Harvard. Here is found the magnificent Longford Castle, surrounded by the Longford Estate, home of the Earl of Radnor. Many of the families and children living on the Estate were included in our survey. Continuing west we have the villages of Nunton, Odstock, Homington, Coombe Bissett, Stratford Tony, Bishopstone, Croucheston, Stoke Farthing, Broadchalke, West End, Bowerchalke, Ebbesbourne Wake, Alvesdiston, and lastly Berwick St John.

When he retired from politics one time Prime Minister Sir Anthony Eden lived in a small cottage in West End. He later moved to Alvesdiston where he died. The village of Bowerchalke was the home of the late Cecil Beaton, artist and royal photographer. His friend Greta Garbo could often be seen walking through the countryside.

I was the driver for Dr Sommerville and following his retirement continued in the same rôle for Dr Roden and matron McDonald. Families with babies and school children were visited weekly, and village schools throughout the valley were visited each Friday. Information was obtained from the school mistress as to the number of colds among the children during the past week. To maintain this schedule it was necessary to be out two or three times each week, usually after doctor and matron's morning round of the volunteers.

The Village Survey began in the spring of 1949 and continued for about two years during which time on several Saturdays children with colds were ferried to Harvard from the school at Ebbesbourne Wake accompanied by a school mistress or parent. The children mixed with the current Harvard resident volunteers after which they were given tea of sticky cakes and buns, icecream, lemonade, orange squash plus a small gift before returning home. The children when returning to school on the Monday naturally informed their friends of their visit to Harvard — every child in the school reported colds a few days before the next scheduled Saturday visit!

I was naturally interested in the scientific side of the survey, but more so in the countryside, meeting the local people, their lifestyles and listening to their stories of life in the valley during the War. Dr Somerville suggested that I could help in visiting some of the families and so I was instructed on the questions to ask and how to record the answers of the housewife/mother one usually met. Pointing to a thatched cottage Dr Sommerville said "That should be an easy one to start with." Making my way along the path to the front door I passed the time of day with an elderly gent in the garden. After gathering my information from the lady of the house I retraced my footsteps and met the elderly gent who I now knew to be grandad, cleaning a bunch of carrots. He stood up and shouted in my ear. "S'now yow'm worsten yow'm tim." (You know you are wasting your time). "Yow 'ont et celd if yow tak 'is" (W'ont get cold if you take this). A snuff box appeared in one hand, thinking I was to participate I put my hand forward to take a pinch. To my surprise it was pushed away and taking a pinch himself he placed his forefinger and thumb on my nose and shouted "Snef Yad." (Sniff hard). Returning to the car Dr Sommerville with a grin on his face asked how I came with soil on my nose!

We were often out during mealtimes. Matron McDonald always made sure flasks of tea or coffee and sandwiches were taken. I was always fond of these meal breaks, most enjoyable, usually stopping on high ground overlooking the spectacular landscape of the Wiltshire countryside, or perhaps down in the valley by the Ebble stream, walking along its banks, trout spotting. Wherever we were there was always an abundance of

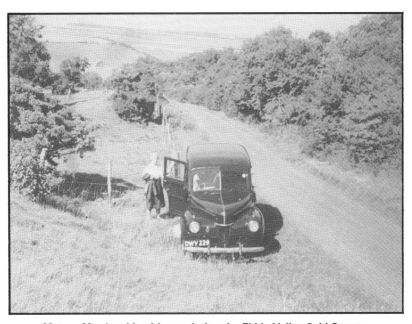

Matron Macdonald, with car, during the Ebble Valley Cold Survey.

birdlife with rabbits and hares together with the odd deer or fox. In spring and early summer the meadows and hedgerows were alive with wild flowers. To my surprise I discovered a small area of wild orchids which I still visit each year when they are in bloom.

The local road repair gang always expected us to stop and pass the time of day, especially as some of their families were taking part in the epidemiological study. The conversation always took on a certain humorous banter and leg pull, so when told smoke was coming from the front passenger door no one took any notice. Eventually we *could* smell burning, and smoke *could* be seen from the outside of the car coming from the bottom of the door panel. The car was a 1937 Austin 10, therefore there was plenty of room to pour a can of water from the roadmen's lorry between the inner and outer door panels. Hot ashes had fallen between these panels when Dr Sommerville knocked his pipe out. Luckily no great damage had been done and we were able to continue our journey.

It was often difficult to get away from some of the more talkative housewives. One would be enlightened as to the families' welfare and also forthcoming village events. Sometimes a hint of scandal would creep in, which was the time to make a diplomatic exit. Many were quite generous with offerings of garden produce and homemade preserves, especially over the Christmas when much stronger beverages were offered, in particular homemade wines.

There was the inevitable guard dog encounter and I remember only one unco-operative, suspicious character who lived at a remote farmhouse.

Through our visits to the villages, long lasting friendships built up with many families. My family and I kept in touch with many after the survey had finished by visiting the village flower shows, fetes and Christmas bazaars. Friends and myself from Salisbury would often visit the village Inns playing darts and skittles with the people we had met during the survey.

Now 40 years on I often meet the school children who came to Harvard those Saturday mornings. They now have children of their own. They still talk of Matron McDonald, who because of her Scottish accent thought she was a sales lady for COAL, not enquiring about COLDS. Also remembering Dr Sommerville and Dr Roden and the Saturday tea parties at Harvard. My wife and I often picnic in those same mealtime stops high on the lonely downs with not a house in sight, only the sound of the skylark, croak of the pheasant with the buzzard soaring over the hills looking for food in the secret valley.

The scientists did not see the Valley as I describe it, but as a statistical analysis and table of figures that school children were mainly responsible for introducing the infection of colds. After all, that is what we went for. Not for me to have a most enjoyable countryside excursion.

Seal Island Colds

Sir Christopher Andrewes mentions in his book *In Pursuit Of The Common Cold* that early attempts to find out how colds passed from one person to another had been frustrated. Evidence of cross-infection had been too infrequent to throw light on the ways in which transmission normally occurred. The volunteers at Harvard seemed to be too resistant. We needed people who might be more susceptible.

It was known that isolated communities often remained free from colds for long periods, until visited by people from the outside world. It occurred to Sir Christopher that it might be possible to find a deserted island where volunteers could live for long enough to lose their resistance and then introduce others with colds, so that cross-infection could be studied. Why not have student volunteers spend their three months summer vacation on such an island? That length of time might be sufficient to render them highly susceptible. The Medical Research Council Air Hygiene Unit was very interested in the possibility that we might solve some of our problems by such a scheme, in which Dr Lovelock of the Air Hygiene Unit took a prominent rôle.

Sir Christopher records how he approached a Scottish colleague of his, Dr (now Sir Frank) Fraser Darling, to see if he knew of a possible deserted island off the coast of Scotland. He not only knew of one, but was helpful and encouraging in other ways. He mentions that the common cold is a relatively serious illness in the remote parts of the Scottish Highlands, everbody is scared of anyone with a cold for varying reasons. Dr Darling goes on to explain that after seven weeks of isolation on Priest Island he and his party were joined by his son, who had a "sniffle," exactly 48 hours after his arrival we all had the same tremendous cold.

Dr Darling told Sir Christopher of the island called Eilean Nan

Rôn (known as the Island of Seals) lying 1½ miles off Skerray, a small fishing village on the north coast of Sutherlandshire. The inhabitants of the island all left in 1938 as they could no longer make a living there, and the younger members of the community would not stay. It contained a number of good houses which might not need much in the way of repair.

The Island belonged to the Duke of Sutherland and after the question of feasibility had been studied and the agreement of the Medical Research Council had been obtained, a letter was sent to the Duke. He gave his consent to our occupying the Island for three months. In May 1950 Sir Christopher Andrewes and Dr Tom Sommerville then the Medical Superintendent at Harvard visited the Island to explore possibilities in more detail.

Eilean Nan Rôn was approximately 1½ miles wide by 2¾ miles long, surrounded by rocky cliffs, and there was a useful jetty with steps leading up the cliffs to a plateau. This was covered with heather and very boggy in places. A well, fed by a spring of good water which had never been known to run dry existed adjacent to the nearest house by the jetty steps.

Sheep grazed amongst the heather, they were tended from time to time by their owners who came over by motor boat from Skerray. Seas were often rough and the journey was usually only possible every other day.

There were 11 houses plus a school house. They were all in good condition, with one exception which had a leaking roof. Some windows were broken, most houses were two up and two down with an outhouse for storage and a copper for washing. Even after 12 years some furniture still remained such as chests of drawers, kitchen dressers and chairs. All were usable after cleaning and a few minor repairs. An ancient mangle was also found later and brought into service.

It was decided that if we could get 12 volunteers to join the expedition we could make eight of the houses habitable, two volunteers in each of six houses using the other two, one which had been the school for a mess, cooking and central services. No water sanitation existed, deep trench and bucket latrines would have to be provided. Opinion was divided on the question of fuel for cooking, we were informed that the peat on the island was of superior quality to that on the mainland. The party could cut their own. However, paraffin was the initial form of heating and cooking. It all looked feasible.

Professor J. S. Young of the Pathology Department at the Aberdeen University persuaded nine students from his department to take part as volunteers. One other came from London — Sir Christopher's son — making up the 12 volunteers was an ex Police Superintendent Mr E. J. Betteridge and his wife Ethel who would be responsible for the party. Mr and Mrs Betteridge did an excellent job, the project was fortunate to have them. It was through their daughter Josephine, a laboratory technician at Harvard, that they were recruited for the job. Mrs Betteridge did all the cooking, which included making the bread with much success.

As mentioned Sir Christopher was a keen entomologist, also Mr Betteridge was interested in ornithology, as was Dr Pennie a doctor on the mainland who was helpful in many ways. He provided rings for ringing sea birds. It seemed the Island party would be useful for biological studies as well as medical research.

A suggestion had been made that stores should be transported from the south to Eilean Nan Rôn by boat. Dr Sommerville decided that with the bad storms "Eilean" was often cut off and stores should be mobilised at Harvard and transported by road to Skerray. A local fisherman — Mr Anderson — an unforgettable character, a man born of the sea was signed on to transport personnel and stores from Skerray to the island. It was important that stores be packed in small lots, for easy loading onto the boat and off loading on the island jetty. Twenty tonnes in all had to be carried up the steep steps in the side of the cliff and then on to the houses.

A Nissen building was set aside at Harvard for the assembly of the island stores which came from three sources — Harvard, RAF and Royal Navy. Harvard supplied blankets, bed linen, towels, crockery, cutlery, and kitchen utensils also folding chairs and some small tables, spades, forks, picks, the latter for latrine and gardening use. From the RAF Institute of Aviation and Medicine came camping equipment, small hospital bedside

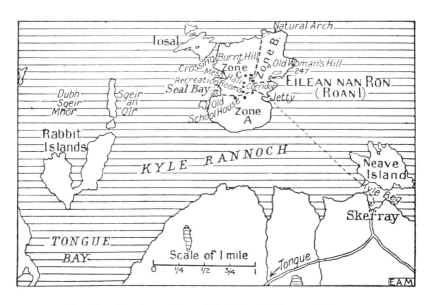

Map showing the position of the Island Of Seals off Skerray.

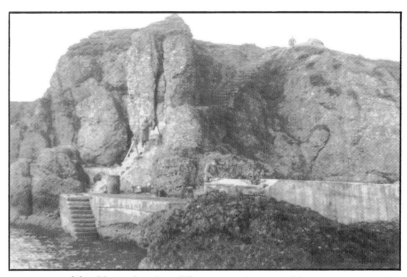

Island jetty showing cliff steps to plateau and houses.

units and collapsible tables and beds, medical equipment and supplies to cover any emergencies.

To get the best buy for food stocks it was decided to approach the victualling department of the Royal Navy. Because of food rationing authorization had to be given by the Ministry of Food, which gave the Island Scheme its blessing. The amount of food was for 13 weeks for 12 people plus two weeks for six extra people. This in food rationing terms added up to 168 man weeks. Of course the island party would have to surrender their ration books. I remember collecting these supplies from the Naval Stores at Portsmouth and when unloading at Harvard it was discovered that butter had not been listed. A further trip to Portsmouth completed the stores. It was discovered much later after the island party had settled in that pepper had been forgotten. All foodstuffs were tinned, including meats, fats, butter, sausages, bacon and of course powdered milk, potatoes by ½ cwt sacks. There were also fresh apples and oranges, the latter which had just become available. Flour was not rationed so plenty was available for baking. Volunteers could not have daily shopping as at Harvard and were therefore asked to bring plenty of cigarettes and tobacco and writing materials for those who intended to continue their university studies. Some cigarettes were taken to sell on the basis of 60 per person per week. A free issue of beer and cider was taken based on ½ pint per person per day. I believe much of this was saved for a binge on the last few days on the Island.

Two Valor oil ranges were taken, as one could not be certain of the efficiency of the old kitchen ranges left behind in many of the houses, or of the peat supplies. Also on the list were six primus stoves, three bungalow baths, six water butts, eight tilley lamps, drums of paraffin for cooking and lighting, slab wood, nails, screws and, of course, basic carpenter's tools for repairs, plus ropes and a wheel-barrow.

Welfare items such as cricket gear, footballs, rugby balls, playing cards, dominoes, chess, dart boards and darts were taken together with two battery operated radios and four radio transmitting and receiving sets. Two sets were housed on the Island and two in the Skerray Shop, these being for the important twice daily radio communications and also allowed for a spare set of equipment at either end. The mainland radio was operated by Miss Jenny McKay, the storekeeper's daughter.

Dr Sommerville made arrangements for billeting the advance party, i.e. Mr and Mrs Betteridge, the volunteer from London and myself. Skerray being a wee "dry" village meant that they were hesitant about taking visitors, one dear lady when asked to take lodgers said "They don't take the drink do they? Because anyone that does will not cross the threshold of my door." The folk I stayed with did take the odd wee dram.

Radio communication was at set times. In case of an emergency it was arranged for a smoke screen by day and Very light at night. Dr Pennie was extremely keen to help and would be only too willing to cope with any emergency should it arise. He also said he was sowing some lettuce seed for planting out on the Island.

The advance party of Dr Sommerville, Dr Lovelock from the Air Hygiene Unit and myself drove up from Harvard in the American estate car, arriving on 27 June 1950 with various pieces of equipment plus tools and materials to carry out minor repairs to the houses on the island. Mr and Mrs Betteridge travelled up by train, the 20 tonnes of stores and equipment arriving by road on Sunday 2 July.

The food and equipment were stored overnight in the outhouse next to Mr McKay's Hardware Shop and the next three days were spent ferrying everything over to the Island. This was very hard work. Luckily we had good weather with fairly calm crossings. Unloading on the Island was often tricky, but thanks to Mr Anderson's experience in handling the boat there were no mishaps.

Carrying 20 tonnes of stores up the cliff face steps onto the plateau and then on to the houses was hard going, but then after all, the people that had lived on the island had to use these steps for taking not only their supplies but also their sheep up and down, so why not us? We used ropes to pull up the drums of paraffin and any other heavy items. I spent most of these days repairing the windows in the houses that were to be used by the

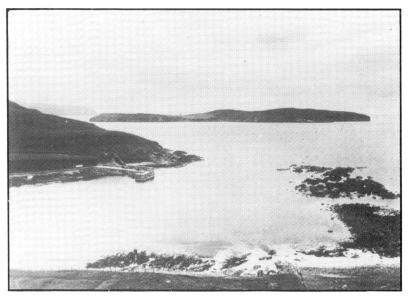

Skerray quay with the Island Of Seals in the background.

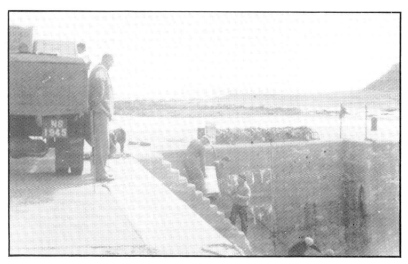

Loading stores at Skerray during lowtide.

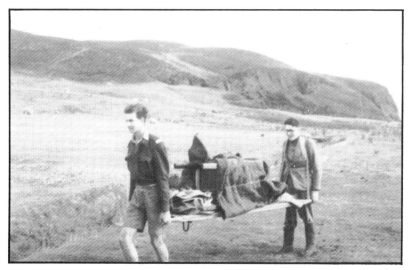

Conveying stores from top of cliff steps to the houses.

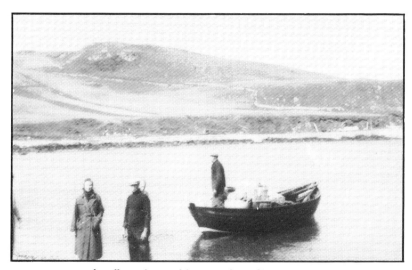

Loading a boat with stores from Skerray quay.

party.

The sun shone until midnight and it remained daylight until the early hours of the morning enabling Mr Anderson and myself to do some sea fishing.

I conveyed the first students from the University of Aberdeen on 6 July, that being the first night that the party slept on the Island. Mr and Mrs Betteridge had worked hard in preparing the mess facilities.

The return jouney to Aberdeen was made the next day to complete the volunteer complement. Mr and Mrs Betteridge, their daughter Josephine, son-in-law Desmond, Dr Sommerville, Dr Lovelock, volunteers and myself spent the next two days making sure that everything was in working order and in its right place. A careful check was made on the Island to Mainland Radio to ensure that it was fully operational. The island at this time was invaded by journalists. Articles appeared not only in the Scottish papers but nationwide with a variety of headlines: "Forbidden Land to all but 12," "Ex City Police Officer in charge of Cold Island," "Exploring Tissue Island," "Seals Trying to Catch Colds," "Sneezing with the Seals on Their Island."

On 11 July Dr Lovelock made the final check of the radio link with the mainland. Mrs Betteridge wrote in her diary "Close Down Island," and appointed her first two kitchen orderlies, Ron and Eric. She also mentions that sea conditions were rough for the following week and that no crossing could be made. We had been very lucky in getting everything over to the island on time.

The first letters from the volunteers to near relatives informing them that all was well were transmitted to Jenny who manned her set at the same time each day, writing out letters and posting them on. Jenny also received weekly newsletters from Mr Betteridge which she phoned direct to Dr Sommerville at Harvard, who in turn had them typed and circulated to the Islanders' nearest relatives. Jenny would inform the island party when owners of the island sheep would be visiting their flock, this would enable them to leave letters at the central point for mailing from the mainland.

The following are extracts from newsletters sent to the relatives from Dr Sommerville that gave them some idea of life on Eilean Nan Rôn (The Island of Seals):—

Newsletter No. 1, dated 21 July 1950

Explains to relatives the radio communication system between mainland and island, the letters to the island should be posted to Jenny at the Skerray Harbour Shop. It goes on to say that everyone is in extremely good spirits in spite of bad weather. Furthermore that they have managed to make themselves very comfortable in the island houses. A number of the party had been fishing with success. The hens which they had taken with them had produced 34 eggs in one week, which they were very pleased with, cockerels were also taken as a source of fresh meat.

Newsletter No. 2, dated 27 July 1950

Begins by reporting that all are in good health. Food ration scales have not been exceeded and that supplies would appear to be ample with the hens having supplemented the stocks with 68 eggs and two non-producers found their way into the pot. The weather had been bright with very heavy storms during Friday and Saturday. The first laundry day had been Wednesday with all work completed by mid-day.

A cricket match was held on Wednesday between Team A captained by Shillingford and Team B captained by Betteridge. The result was a draw. Top scorer for Team A was Shillingford with 21 and for Team B — Betteridge also 21. Team B are supplying the umpire and scorers for the next match. A win for Team B is expected.

Three of the party crossed to the adjoining island of Eilean Josel. Crossing is difficult but safe at low tide. An expedition is planned for all on the next suitable tide.

Fishing had been poor with the lobster pots producing nothing edible.

The camp carpenter, John Matthews, had now completed his handiwork and general states of fatigue had finished.

Also a great interest had been taken in birdwatching. Several

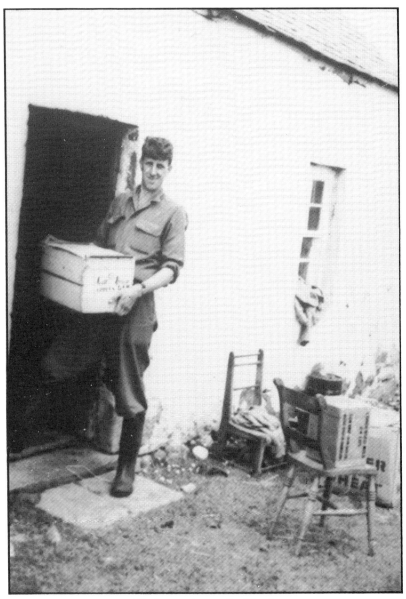

Storing apples on the Island.

birds having been ringed with the rings supplied by Dr Pennie.

Newsletter No. 3, dated 2 August 1950
The report opens with the news that all are in good health and free from colds. Food supplies were ample, the hens had produced 64 eggs and that bread making was so far proving to be a great success. Weather had remained unsettled with Sunday having been a particularly bad day.

Again the week had been a quiet one. The island provided such a variety of interests that there was never a dull moment. Study takes up a considerable part of the students' time, but there is a little sport thrown in at times. The cricket match had again resulted in a draw despite the efforts of the scorer, a member of Team B.

Fishing was again poor, and they had not been able to catch sufficient bait for the lobster pots. They offered no excuses except that the winds and tides were really useless.

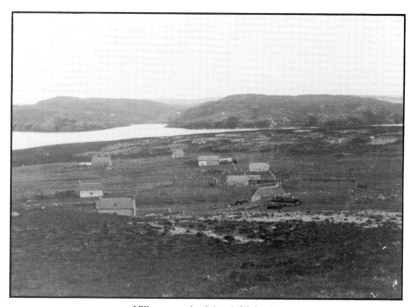

Village on the Island Of Seals.

Newsletter No. 4, dated 10 August 1950
Health remains excellent with no colds. Food rations remained ample dispite the healthy appetites. The supplies of fruit and vegetables had kept amazingly well. The hens had produced 61 eggs during the week. Weather conditions had improved, they had had several very good days.

A planned expedition to Eilean Josel took place on Friday. They crossed at 8.00 am taking with them food and drink for the day. After exploring the island they searched for Stormy Petrels and were successful in finding a large number. They managed to ring 20 Stormy Petrels, also four gulls and six shags. The return to Eilean Nan Rôn was at 8.30 in the evening with everyone having agreed it had been a glorious day.

Saturday was John Wilson's birthday and they celebrated with a large iced cake for afternoon tea.

A favourable report for fishing was anticipated for the following week.

Newsletter No.5, dated 17 August 1950
Everyone still remained in good health and free from colds.

After five weeks of careful rationing it was now clear that there were sufficient stocks to see them through to the end of the trial. However, they would probably appreciate a few smaller items when the Medical Team joined them in September, but it was not anticipated that the order would be a large one. They were working up a reserve which should give them ample quantities of basic items for the last 14 days with an additional small reserve in case of emergencies. The egg production for the week had fallen to only 29.

The weather had been unsettled with very high winds and some rain most days. In fact the weekly cricket match on Wednesday had been stopped for bad weather! However, it is an ill wind that blows nobody any good, the students had a very good week for studying.

The garden which had been omitted from previous reports showed considerable promise until the current week when high winds and a raid by birds played havoc with the lettuce plants.

Serious fishing had not been possible during the week owing

to high winds and rough sea — better luck for the following week?

Newsletter No.6, dated 24 August 1950
General health remained excellent and still no colds. Rations remained the same with the addition of a few radishes from the garden and egg production had risen to 34. The weather had been variable, wet and cold. The worst week so far.

During the week the island had been visited by the owners of the sheep. There had been no contact with them. To their knowledge no-one else had attemped to land there, but the passing fishing boats generally gave a call on their sirens. A most fearsome looking gallows had been erected in full view of the quay together with a notice which should be sufficient to keep anyone away.

A very large fish, said to be a shark, had been seen on several occasions close to the shore. Judging by the estimate as to its size it appeared to be growing at an alarming rate.

During Saturday night and Sunday morning there had been a wonderful cascade of the Northern Lights owing to the bad weather.

Exchange rates had remained steady but it would not be a surprise if the value of cigarettes increased.

Fishing had again been poor and it would appear that it was impossible to compete against sharks, seals and Mr Anderson!

Newsletter No.7, dated 31 August 1950
Another healthy cold free week with unsettled weather and egg production down to 12.

For 3½ days during the week everyone lived in their own houses as a rehearsal for the last fortnight of isolation. Everyone enjoyed the change, especially the weekly kitchen orderlies. All fed surprisingly well thanks to the large pies and tarts provided by Mrs Betteridge. During those few days various culinary experiments took place.

Party A had fried bread, bacon and eggs for the first home-made breakfast. However after burning the bread and bacon they lost heart and decided to save their eggs for another meal. Three members of the party declared that condensed milk made excellent toffee. The cook has yet to discover what happened to his only tin!

With Party B it was a case of too many cooks. Their decision to use their curried dumplings as cricket balls was not accepted as the cricket bat was falling to pieces. To increase their egg supplies they lured the hens into their outhouse — to the depletion of their stock of Army Biscuits. The hens however remained loyal to House 2 and went home to lay.

Party C seized the opportunity to utilise their extra culinary skills and indulged in some luxurious living. Their fudge was very good but had a tendency to smell. A new recipe was discovered which was far too complicated for inclusion in a newsletter.

The reopening of the communal kitchen was celebrated with the last of the potatoes (four cheers from the four kitchen orderlies!) and three chickens — blissful groans of indigestion.

A fishing net had been constructed which yielded 15 saithe and two shags. This poaching method was scorned by the purist exponents of the rod and line. Gour had caught 18 saithe but no shags. The poachers watched anxiously in case the fishery cruiser should find the net within the three mile coast boundary. It was now certain that there were two sharks in local waters. The lobster pots had produced one good sized crab and the first lobster 1ft 5ins long.

The owners of the sheep had been again and taken away some lambs to Skerray. There had been no contact with them.

Bird life had become more interesting, particularly with the small land birds which were congregating ready for migration.

It was possible that this message had been altered and extended by one wireless operator and further mutilated by another.

Newsletter No.8, dated 6 September 1950
Still no colds and excellent health with food rations still ample. There was an improvement in the weather which had allowed for sunbathing and some glorious sunsets.

Fishing had shown an improvement. The lobster pots had

yielded a further lobster and large crab. Three fairly large dog-fish were also caught (one of them in the lobster pot) and used for bait in other pots. Winkles had featured on the menu for the first time. The sharks had been seen again several times and one evening when some of the party were fishing from the quay one passed within a few feet of them forcing them to pull in their lines. The estimated length of the shark was 20 ft.

Thursday's cricket match had resulted in a win for Team A by one run.

The heather was now in full bloom covering most of the island. A check of the Stormy Petrels' nests was being carried out for Dr Pennie and to date 21 nests had been discovered.

Mrs Betteridge entered in her diary each day's menu, for example on Friday 21 July, seven days into isolation period:—

Breakfast

> Porridge or cereal, boiled eggs, bread, butter and jam.

Lunch

> Herrings in tomato sauce, cheese, bread and apples.

Dinner

> Soup, beef steaks, carrots, boiled onions, potatoes, rice pudding and coffee.

The menu on Friday 25 August — 40 days into the island isolation period:—

Breakfast

> Bacon, sausage, fried potatoes, jam, marmalade, bread and butter.

Lunch

> Corned beef, potato chips, apple crumble and cream, bread and butter.

Dinner

> Three chickens — suspect non-layers — potatoes,

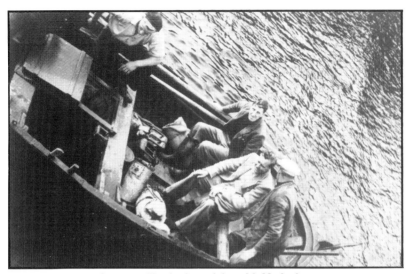

Dr Sommerville sharing a joke with Mr Anderson.

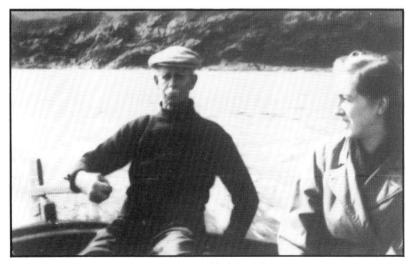

Mr Anderson with Josephine.

peas, gravy, peaches and custard, coffee.

Supper

Bread, butter, jam, meat paste, biscuits and tea.

The last full menu for Monday 2 October read:—

Breakfast

Porridge and cereal, boiled eggs, bread, butter and marmalade.

Lunch

Soup, corned beef, potatoes, cabbage, salad, cheese and biscuits. (Cabbage we suspect had been taken over by the scientists when they went to collect fresh vegetables).

Dinner

Roast chicken, peas, potatoes, gravy, pears, peaches and cream, coffee.

Supper

Bread, butter, jam and tarts.

When one remembers that there was no electricity supply for the use of refrigerators Mrs Betteridge did extremely well.

A good description of life on the island is given by Mr J. Davidson — a member of the party of 12 volunteers. He begins by saying that he and his companions volunteered to go to Rôn Island because they felt that it was a chance of a lifetime to have a cheap, but unusual holiday.

We had been told that there were fine opportunities not only for fishing, swimming and bird watching but also for uninterrupted study. The real attraction however was to be able to get away from the drab routine of urban life. When we landed on Rôn we found the houses to be in amazingly good condition, all being wind and waterproof, each one of us had our own room and there was a wireless receiver for each house, which proved to be our only source of entertainment and contact with the outside world.

A rota of orderlies was drawn up to help Mr and Mrs Betteridge who had volunteered to be temporary *father and mother* to us. Cooking was done on paraffin stoves, once a week the kitchen was converted into a bakehouse where bread was successfully made. (The island bread was so successful that when Mr and Mrs Betteridge returned home they did not like their baker's bread and carried on making their own. It was never the same as that made on the island, Mrs Betteridge said that it was due to the island's spring water.) Mrs Betteridge kept us well supplied with baked goodies, even an iced birthday cake was provided inspite of the lack of facilities.

Our fishermen had some unforgettable experiences whilst fishing from the rocks near the jetty. Fish caught were mostly saithe and dog fish but on one occasion a 40lb anglia fish was lined. One memorable night a shoal of fish entered the inlet with the water boiling with jumping fish, followed by a large Atlantic seal, which after eating its fill lay grunting with satisfaction on the rocks nearby.

Bottles containing messages were thrown into the sea, one reaching Stronsay beach, Orkney, and a second Scrabster, near John O'Groats. A reply to the first was received within two weeks.

As the summer passed the weather grew worse, gales and rain forcing us to spend most of our time indoors reading and studying or listening to the wireless.

Many evenings were spent around a roaring peat and wood fire playing bridge, having long discussions or singing to the accompaniment of the guitar and mouth organ. Our wireless sets kept us right with the time and day of the week, which was of little significance to us that it was frequently forgotten. Thanks mainly to the efficient planning and the selection of this ideal island we were all agreed that this had been the most unusual and enjoyable holiday spent for the cost of *one common cold*.

It was planned that some of the volunteers would vacate the island on Monday 2 October, however the seas became too rough for the crossing to be made. The following day Sir Christopher and Dr Lovelock did make it over to the island and some of the volunteers crossed back to the mainland.

On Wednesday 4 October the island was again invaded by jounalists, talking to everyone and gathering material for their respective papers. Mr and Mrs Betteridge together with the rest of the volunteers left the island and were put up at the small hotel at Borgie, a village about three miles from Skerray. A dance was held that evening in the village hall, instigated I suspect by Dr Pennie for all the villagers and boatmen that took part in the island scheme, the little hut was full, the whole village came. Music was provided by the volunteers' guitar and mouth organ, plus a boatman with his accordian. There was no bar, but for a *dry* village with no pub it was miraculous how the whisky appeared, and then disappeared down upturned throats.

The following seven days were spent bringing remaining stores and equipment from the island, all the houses being left in good order.

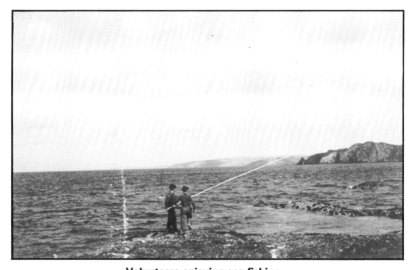

Volunteers enjoying sea fishing.

As for myself I spent the week conveying the volunteers back to their homes or to the University of Aberdeen. The journey from Skerray to Aberdeen was approximately 180 miles. There were no motorways or dual carriageways. Much of the road from Skerray to Inverness was single track with passing places. The overnight stops were sometimes with Dr Sommerville's parents in Aberdeen or bed and breakfast. On one occasion I attempted the round trip in one day but finished sleeping in the estate car when fog closed in.

It was during this time when out fishing late one evening with Mr Anderson that the *Aurora Borealis* was displaying overhead. A most memorable fishing trip.

Sir Christopher Andrewes stated that it was one of the most glamorous experiments in which he had ever been engaged.

The Island Experiment was not put on for me to tour Scotland, to go sea fishing, or enjoy a dram with the folk with whom I lodged. Sir Christopher Andrewes, Dr Sommerville and Dr Lovelock spent long hours conducting a series of cold trials. It was hoped that the 12 inhabitants of the island, had acquired by virtue of their isolation a susceptibility to colds greater than they would have if they had been living in a large community. The plan was to divide the islanders into three entirely separate parties as explained in newsletter No. 7 when the Island party had had a three day rehearsal for the final two weeks of the experiment.

Now came the time to test this susceptibility to colds. As mentioned the islanders were divided into three parties *A, B, C* for whom contact would be made in three different ways. The island was also divided into three different zones, with each party keeping within its own zone. They also had, of course, to cook for themselves.

On 19 September Sir Christopher Andrewes and Dr Lovelock arrived and joined party C to discover if people not having colds could possibly be carrying viruses which could be passed on. Late on 23 September Dr Sommerville landed with five additional students I had brought from Aberdeen University, who had colds. All six had been inoculated with cold virus from laboratories at Harvard, and fortunately all had developed

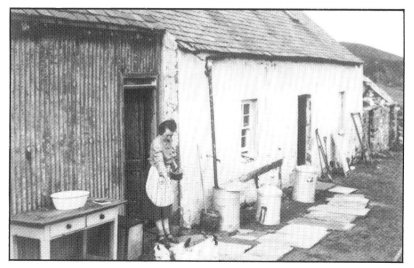

Feeding time for the hens.

colds. Crucial experiments began and continued until 3 am the next morning.

First party *A* left their house which was then occupied for three hours by the six people with colds. They played cards, handled the cutlery, books and anything that laid around. The cold carriers then left and the house was re-occupied by party *A*. The object was to see whether colds could be transferred by handling infected objects.

The six colds then moved to a separated room in party *B*'s house, this was divided by a blanket partition not quite reaching the floor or ceiling. This was to establish whether small particles and droplets would pass from one side of the room to the other with the six colds on one side of the blanket and party *B* on the other. Those with colds coughed, sneezed and talked throughout the three hours and then left.

Lastly party *C* lived and ate with the cold sufferers for three days. To the scientists' astonishment and dismay not a single cold developed among the 12 islanders.

A few days later another party of four students arrived with the Harvard infected colds, again no colds developed despite close contact with the islanders. Was it possible that the so called *pedigree colds* from Harvard had lost the power to pass from one person to another even though they produced when dropped up the subjects noses.

Sir Christopher heard through the radio of a crofter on the mainland who had a good cold, he was persuaded to make a day trip to the island and stayed talking round the fire for about four hours to the island volunteers. His cold was passed its prime, having begun five days before, nevertheless four out of the 12 islanders developed colds. It was interesting to note that I spent five to six hours in an enclosed vehicle when driving cold sufferers from Aberdeen to Skerray without so much as a sniffle.

The Island Experiment was not, as it seems a failure. It was, with the *Ebble Valley — An Epidemiology Study* combining with this and the Harvard Ten Day Volunteer Trials giving the scientists information on how the viruses were transmitted. Remember this was 1950 when very little was known on the subject.

The final evacuation of the island took place on Friday 6 October when the Island seals returned to a solitude, broken only by the cry of the sea birds.

The last crossing to the mainland was very rough with heavy seas running in the Kyle of Ronnoch. I drove the estate car to the end of the harbour for loading the last odds and ends from the boat. The wind felt like a dagger's point, chilling the skin, and I thought that the cold for some time would be a common hazard on life.

My wife and I returned to the Skerray Harbour in 1984 and sadly saw that tragedy had overtaken two members of Mr Anderson's boat crew of 1950, for at the end of the harbour wall was in inscribed plaque which read, *In memory of Hector McKay and John Anderson, lost at sea in 1973 while fishing.*

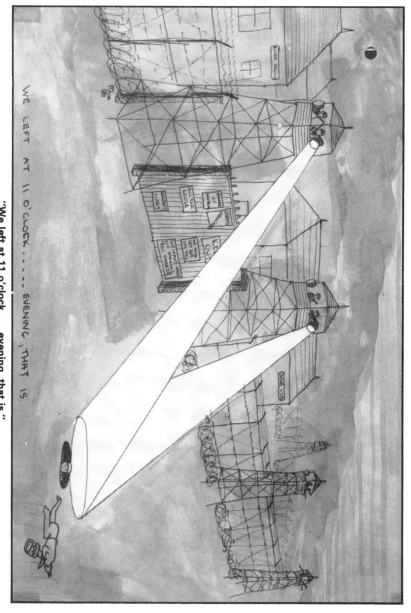

"We left at 11 o'clock . . . . evening, that is."

Reflections

I did not find the work at Harvard irksome or tedious. There was always plenty of scope for inventiveness. The laboratory scientist would, from time to time make changes to the trial routine, many of them at very short notice, perhaps even needing to alter the layout to the volunteer living accommodation.

With the Common Cold Unit's use of volunteers being unique there was no means of referment for guidance. Here was a small unit where all aspects of administration were dealt with in one office.

All the work carried out by the administration was of a supportive rôle to the laboratory staff and scientists, enabling them to get the best from the volunteers in the time available. The Monday to Friday 9 am to 5 pm was out of the question. All the volunteers were in residence for ten days round the clock. Matron was on continuous duty during this time and sometimes needed some support, as did the night watchman.

Overseas scientists from India, Japan, China, America, Norway, Sweden, Russia, Venezuella, Brazil and Europe took up much of the administrative time. Some stayed a few weeks or months, whilst others remained for one or two years. Most of the scientists required accommodation at Harvard. Those staying for long periods would often ask for assistance in a variety of ways, for example buying a car, banking facilities, provision of a family doctor and so on. Those married with children required help in finding suitable schools. One delightful eight year old American deaf and dumb girl went to the local village school at Odstock and made better strides in communications than at home in the "States."

Several Russian scientists came, all of whom were very pleasant and extrovert in their ways. One of their party could not understand why volunteers came of their own freewill.

Another, an amorous type, was always with a lady friend. I shall always remember taking one lady to the station where she promptly burst into a flood of tears, not wanting to board the train. Eventually by half carrying and half dragging her I managed to get her to her seat on the train.

Harvard had many distinguished visitors during its War years, many well known screen stars, high ranking Service Officers including General Eisenhower. Yehudi Menuhin gave a concert here. The late Queen Mary paid a visit and during her tour of the unit was asked if she would like to use the ladies room (specially prepared) but Her Majesty declined the offer. The tour continued but a short time later she requested the use of same in another building which she was passing. After her return home to nearby Bathampton her lady in waiting wrote expressing her gratitude, also mentioning that the Union Jack had been flown upside down!

Many volunteers asked if we had a room set aside as a private place of worship and meditation. One was never provided and it has always been regretted that this was not done.

Mr Waltho, the first permanent Administrator, decided that the unit should be self sufficient and grow its own vegetables since there was plenty of spare ground. In my capacity as driver I was given the job of ploughman and for hours attemped to steer a straight furrow with the most atrocious piece of mechanism I have ever handled. It consisted of two iron wheels and a single cylinder engine — which untied one's bootlaces every time it fired. Attempting to keep the single ploughshare at a constant depth and on a straight course was near impossible. Vegetable growing was short lived.

Providing and maintaining the volunteers' part time amenities needed constant attention, but they did help to achieve a good volunteer relationship. Some people even came during the summer months especially to play croquet.

Matron Margaret Andrews began an excellent amenity, namely the Harvard scrapbook for volunteers to record their comments. These books were in constant use, and 15 years on when the unit closed there were six volumes full of entertaining reading, with photographs and many cartoons.

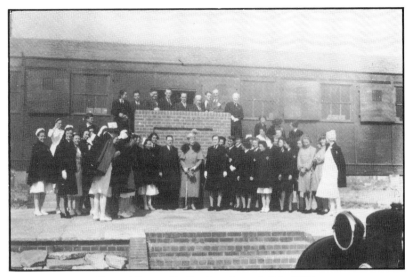

Queen Mary with the American staff in 1944.

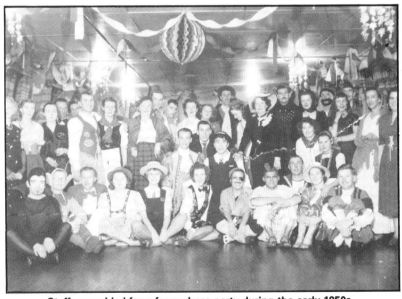

Staff assembled for a fancy dress party during the early 1950s.

During the War the American Red Cross had a store in London supplying rehabilitation handicrafts and games to their British and European hospitals. When this store closed much of the supplies were sent to Harvard for volunteers to use.

We often had visits from ex-Wartime staff from the "States," showing great interest and always surprised that the Old Unit was still thriving.

Reunions of Wartime staff took place in America with two held at Harvard in 1964 and the second in 1989 when 16 of the 55 remaining members of the original staff attended.

A special dedication service was held in Salisbury Cathedral to honour the six nurses who were lost at sea when their ship was torpedoed crossing the Atlantic. This service was followed by a visit to Harvard for a final look round and tea. Polly Kuehnert an original staff nurse summed up the occasion by

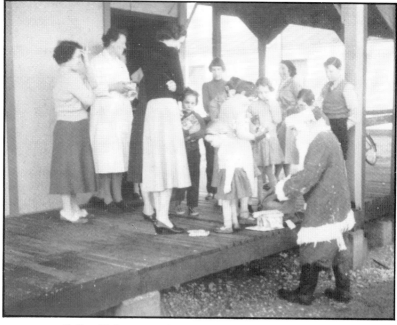

Father Christmas paying a visit to the resident families.

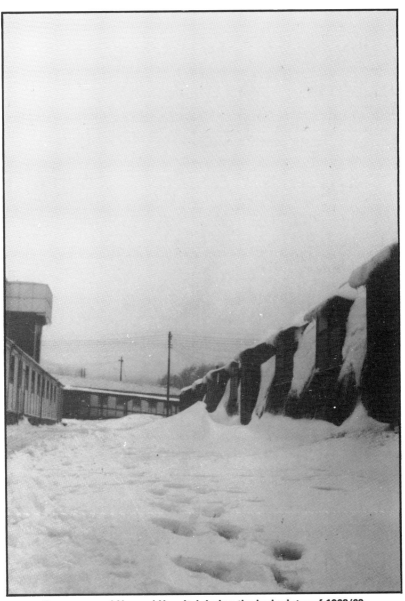

Snow covered Harvard Hospital during the bad winter of 1962/63.

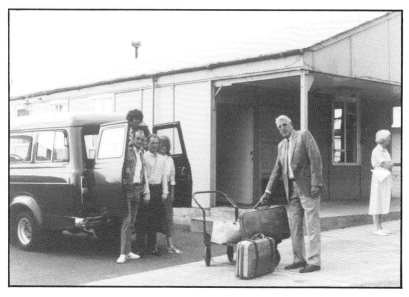

27 July 1989 — Farewell to the last of Harvard's volunteers.

saying "We were here to open Harvard and again to close it." On 4 July 1989, the American celebration of Independence Day, it was fitting with the forthcoming closure of Harvard that the Harvard Trainer aircraft, from the Second War should fly over the unit dipping it's wings in salute to it's twin.

The gale force winds of 25 January 1990 demolished most of the connecting walkways, causing iron roof sheeting to crash into the building panels, exposing the interiors to the mercy of the heavy rain. Which seemed that perhaps the "final curtain" was not that of Man.

Buildings And Their Upkeep

The Harvard site covered 15½ acres and consisted of 40 buildings of three different structures, 21 of which were 120ft long and 20ft wide and housed patient wards, plus doctors' and nurses' living quarters, laboratories, laundry, kitchen and dining room, finally a building that the Americans called the "Club House." Transported over with these buildings were connecting 4ft wide wooden slatted walkways covered by corrugated iron sheet similar to sidewalks seen in American westerns. Eight smaller buildings, 62ft by 8 ft, built on a concrete base, were situated on the right hand side of the driveway coming in through the main entrance and used for men's living quarters. These could serve no useful purpose to the Common Cold Unit so they were demolished shortly after our arrival. Finally there were 10 Nissen buildings of varying sizes. The three larger ones were used as a medical school and lecture room, the second for administration and the third as store and blood bank detachment supply. Harvard Blood Bank played an important part during the Normandy landings.

The remaining Nissens were used for sanitation, showers, a boiler house with two close to the main gate used as men's dining room and cookhouse. An animal house and stores completed the Nissen complex. A further 12 buildings of brick construction were the boiler houses, main gate guard room, the garage, four air raid shelters, electrical transformer house, plus a building containing boiler house and showers which were never used as they were equipped for personal decontamination in the event of a gas attack. This was well appointed with an array of showers. Two 25,000 gallon water tanks supported on large brick plinths have proved to be a land mark for Harvard. The water passing through a softening plant

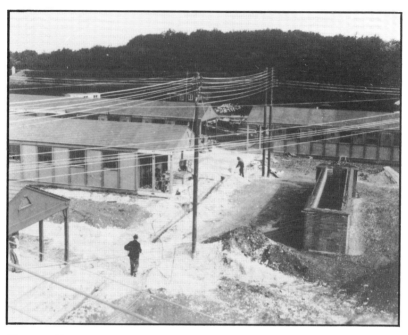

**Above and below: The Common Cold Research Unit, during construction, in 1941
(photographs courtesy of Mrs Lois M. Simon).**

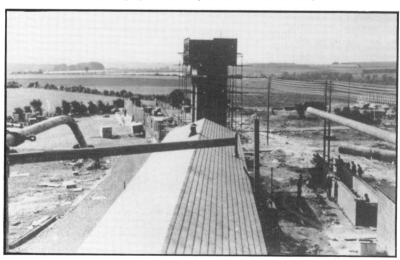

situated near the back gate.

With so much wooden construction Harvard was a high fire risk, but had good fire prevention facilities. There were four fire hydrants from the main water supply. The two water towers could also be used. There were also three static tanks sunk 60ft into the ground and water from these tanks could be pumped by Harvard's own high powered fire trailer housed in the garage building. These tanks were eventually filled in and the trailer dispensed with.

For convenient transportation from the USA all 21 main buildings were of prefabricated structure, the exterior wall panels measuring 8ft by 4ft of weatherproof material with roughly every third panel fitted with a window of wire reinforced glass and fitted with an anti-fly screen. The interior partitioning panels were of plywood and the same size, the 4ft by 4ft ceiling panels were also plywood. Flooring was 1in. plywood with both sides being oak faced. The under floor joists and roof supports being 10in wide and 1in. thick planking doubled and held together by 3in spacers. Both roof and floor supports were placed 4ft apart along the full length of the building. The floor joists were secured to 12ins square base timbers or so called sole plates supported from the ground by square concrete uprights.

The support structure looked much like farm buildings which stand on staddle stones. Under the flooring and above the ceiling panels a lining of wood fibre insulation was laid. There was no plastic foam insulation as we know it today. The roof itself was covered by metal shingles.

The 4ft wide doors made movement of stretchers and furniture very easy. A small viewing window fitted to each of the ward doors enabled the nurse to keep an eye on her patients without entering the ward. The nurse on duty in the wards could be summoned to a patient's bed by a tell tale light above her desk switched on by the patient at the bed head, a light also shone outside the ward, informing her as to where she was required.

Drugs, general store and linen cupboards were situated next to the nurse's desk in the centre of the building. The building consisted of four double and single wards, bathroom, washroom equipped with sterilizing unit and bed pan flush. Door funiture was all solid brass. Corridors in the wards were 8ft wide, i.e. two panels allowing ample room to swing a stretcher. In the nurses' and doctors' living quarters corridors were only one panel wide, giving the advantage of larger rooms.

The doctors' and nurses' living accommodation consisted of nine single bedrooms, two sitting rooms plus a self-contained unit with private bathroom and toilet. Showers, bath and toilet for general use were positioned in the centre of the building.

Each building had its own oil-fired thermostatically controlled central heating and hot water system, the boiler house being centrally positioned. There was a radiator in each room and eight throughout the corridor. The diesel fired boiler was fed by 100 gallon tanks situated outside each boiler room and these tanks were in turn filled by a pump from a 5,000 gallon tank adjacent to the main garage. A second tank was added in 1968 due to industrial action delaying supplies.

The heating and hot water system was well planned and very efficient. All the equipment was manufactured from good quality materials. It was not until after 25 years of continuous use that any of the boilers needed to be replaced, in fact six of the original boilers were still in operation when the Unit closed. A major contribution to their long service was the use of softened water preventing scale forming in the supply pipes and of course the boilers. All water with the exception of that used for drinking passed through a softener benefiting the laundry, laboratories and all washing facilities. The boiler system described was at least 25 years ahead of its time.

The interior of the laboratories were partitioned in much the same way as the staff quarters. Some flooring had to be reinforced to take heavy pieces of laboratory equipment.

The kitchen comprised of two large rooms, plus a spacious dining room. Cooking was done with a diesel oil fired oven. Bread and cake ovens were also oil fired. Steam fed from the laundry heated the boilers cooking the vegetables. These with the bread and cake ovens were removed, the C.C.U. not having

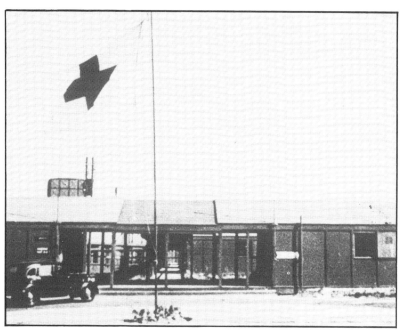

Red Cross flag flying at wartime Reception Area (photograph courtesy of Mrs Lois M. Simon).

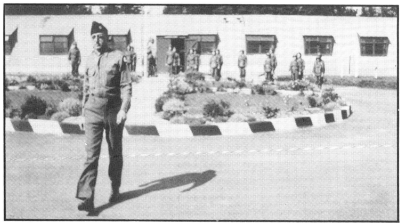

American staff on parade outside the Nissen huts which housed Administration (photograph courtesy of Mrs Lois M. Simon).

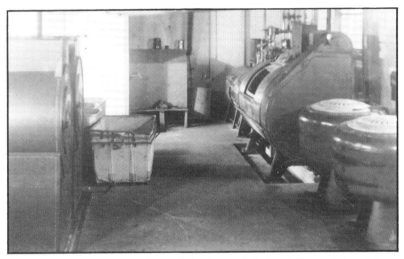

Above and below: Two views of the laundry interior at Harvard Hospital.

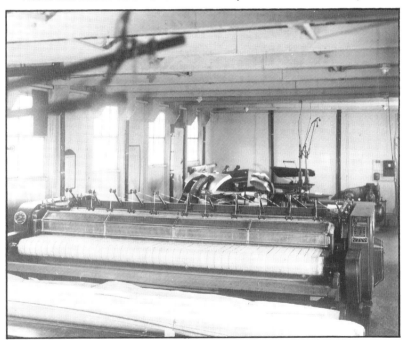

the same large numbers as the Americans to cater for. The walk-in cold room was retained and still being used when the Unit closed.

The laundry was best described to me by Max Kuehnert and his wife Polly during a visit to the Unit in 1977. Polly, who was a nurse from Pennsylvania, came over with the Red Cross to Harvard in 1940. She met Max of the US Army stationed nearby at Longford Castle, in fact he moved in as Field Marshall Montgomery moved out in 1942. They met, courted and became the first American Service couple to wed in Europe during the Second World War. Max and Polly went on to explain how the American Red Cross went to great lengths to obtain the most up to date equipment for the laundry which included the huge oil fired boiler. The laundry became a show piece. So much so that distinguished visitors to the unit during the War were always shown around it.

The Common Cold Unit's limited amount of linen rendered this unit an uneconomical proposition and it was handed over to the local hospital group who continued its operation until 1984, the original equipment lasting for much of that time.

The 240 volt electrical system to the unit passed through a transformer to accommodate the 110 volt American system. From the transformer house the supply passed to each building by overhead cable, which gave problems during severe gales. A change from 110 volt to 240 volt took place in 1949 when all the buildings were re-wired to comply with British safety standards.

Unfortunately, when the buildings were first erected no gutterings were fitted allowing the rain to run down the sides of the buildings soaking into the sole plates and base timbers. It was not until 1952 that guttering was fitted.

The replacement of supporting timbers and the beginning of an ongoing repair programme started in the early 1950s and because the authorities would, or could not make a firm decision as to how long the Common Cold Unit work would continue there was no annual allocation of finance for repair work. This meant that each job had to be negotiated with the responsible bodies i.e. the D.H.S.S. and their building agents the Department of Enviroment (D. of E.).

Not before 1960 did the Harvard administration assess their own estimated expentiture for the following financial year, regarding repairs, new work, furniture, soft furnishings and replacements and general supplies. The D.H.S.S. commissioned the DoE to employ the building contractors and oversee all work. A fee of 30% of all costs being levied to cover their services. This arrangement was not economical for the C.C.U. as it reduced the value of the annual allocation of funds. We were continually fighting red tape and bureaucracy to obtain value for money with little or no success.

The Medical Research Council had from the outset financed the laboratory, office and transport sections and in the mid 1970s they became responsible for all supplies and building repairs. The Harvard administration had full control of their annual allocation of funds. We were then able to save the 30% fee levied by the D. of E. and obtain value for money.

We cannot, when referring to general repairs, forget to mention Mr Alan Brown, affectionately known to all as "Micky." He first came to Harvard in 1948, employed by the contractors. Although not directly employed by the unit Micky stayed for 35 years by switching to each new contractor and finally becoming self-employed. The connecting wooden walkways needed constant attention. Micky's first job each morning being the inspection of same, replacing dangerous slats. By the end of his 35 years all slats and many supporting timbers had been replaced. Over the years he replaced all rotted window frames, cover strips, plus many exterior panels which became cracked and broken due to the decaying base support timbers. These base support timbers were replaced by concrete blocks, thus supporting the full length of the building which no doubt prolonged the life of Harvard.

The re-building of Harvard was talked about for many years, the first meeting took place in 1974. Nothing much more was done until 1979 when the MRC employed architects to draw up necessary plans. I found this a most exciting time attending meetings with Dr Tyrrell and Mrs Brown at MRC Head Office in London until final plans were eventually drawn up. Much work

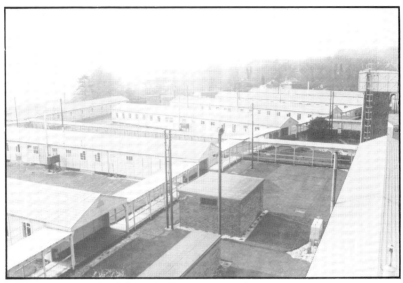

Above and below: The Unit looking in good shape. Two views from the water tower.

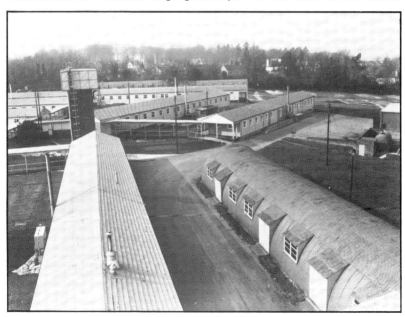

133

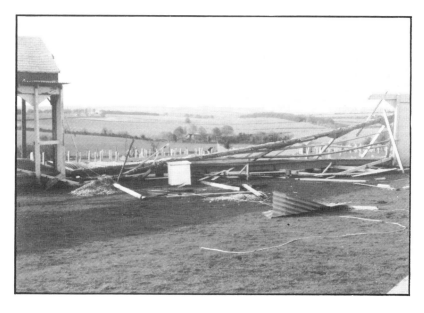

Above and below: Some effects of the gales of January 1990.

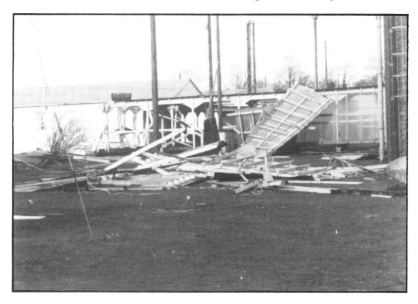

was done by Mrs Brown who planned the new laboratories and myself for volunteer, staff and administration accommodation. The final plans were submitted in 1981. During these planning years with a new building in the pipeline only essential repairs were carried out.

When the decision not to rebuild came in the spring of 1982 poor old Harvard looked much the worse for wear and the decision not to continue with the common cold investigation using volunteers signalled its closing.

The Unit's flower beds and borders and the array of hanging baskets outside the reception area have for many years been Dennis (Mr Clissold's), the Unit groundsman's pride and joy. The well kept lawns between the buildings and the outcrop of closely cut green bordering the boundary fence, the added attraction of the Wiltshire countryside rising and falling in the distance has a pleasant visual impact.

Harvard has been judged the winner of Salisbury's Britain in Bloom Award — Community Group category many times — thanks to Dennis. The appreciation of our groundsman's craft would have had little significance had the grounds not been well landscaped in the first instance.

During its construction Harvard would have looked like any other building site with its mountains of white chalk from the digging of underground services, construction of roadways, excavation of footings and not forgetting the three sunken static tanks each holding 20,000 gallons of water.

One must again remember the shortage of mechanical earth moving equipment. Rationing of fuel meant that most of the landscaping would have had to be done by hand — for this prisoners of war were employed — German or Italian no matter which — they did a magnificent job and we thank them.

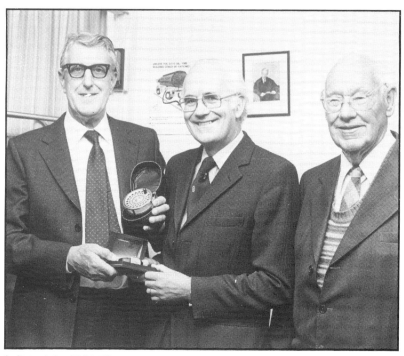

Left to right: Keith Thompson, Dr Tyrrell, and Sir Christopher Andrewes, on the occasion of Keith Thompson's retirement in 1982.

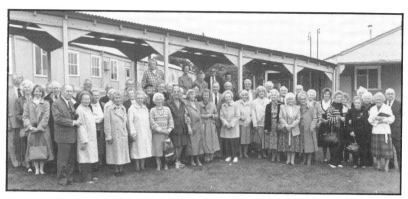

American wartime staff say goodbye on 7 October 1989 (photograph courtesy of the *Salisbury Times And Journal Series***).**

Appendix Two
Both Volunteer And Staff

It is interesting to have the opinion of the Unit from someone who had been both volunteer and a member of staff.

Miss J. Bailey, who came many times as a volunteer first in 1953, joined the staff as Matron in 1970. Her enrolment as a volunteer was the result of the unit's publicity in the national press. It was her natural curiosity for something different and the chance to study for ten days undisturbed in the countryside that prompted her to become a volunteer.

Miss Bailey comments:—

> Amongst my circle of friends it was considered an odd way to spend a holiday, some thought it was quite masochistic, perhaps with youth and good health, one was not worried about anything going wrong, having implicit faith in the medical and scientific staff.

> I was deeply impressed by the superb panoramic views, the freedom to walk miles, knowing good food and comfort was waiting back in the flat. The staff were efficient. There was always a welcome and someone was always on hand to help with individual problems. Routine did not vary greatly from one trial to another, it all seemed rock solid.

> Authority was in evidence, Miss Macdonald, the Matron at the time, was not to be taken lightly, when she entered the flat with her broad Scots accent saying "Now girls." Then we all took notice! A character indeed, but for all her sternness a most comforting person to have around if coughs and sneezes proved irksome.

> There was a degree of camaraderie amongst most volunteers meeting up on the last evening with people from different walks of life, comparing notes on isolation

and other aspects of the trial. These discussions with such a variety of lifestyles and opinions was an education in itself. Many lasting friendships were formed, most of us considered this episode in our lives to be enjoyable and much appreciated.

We were all very hopeful that we would not develop a cold or influenza and were somewhat surprised when we did, but never annoyed. Rather, consolation and a feeling that as an individual you had made a contribution to medical research. The pocket money and the freedom at the end of the trial made one forget any inconvenience and like myself many would volunteer again.

Miss Bailey then talks about Harvard as a member of staff. She first wrote stating that if a matron's post became available she would like to be considered for the vacancy. Shortly after her initial inquiry the post became vacant and Miss Bailey came for an interview. There was not the usual question and answer exchange but a discussion from which it was decided that she should join a forthcoming trial as a volunteer again during which time the Medical Superintendent and myself could meet and get to know her in order to establish that the three post holders could work as a team.

Miss Bailey continues:—

Joining the Unit in March and having been used to working inside I soon felt the wrath of the cold windswept walkways between the flats. I soon settled in realising how fortunate I had been having had the experience of being a volunteer thereby knowing the routine. A question I asked myself was how the scientific staff viewed the volunteers? Were they just an essential part of the trial or were they seen as having individual identities? Because of the smallness of the workforce people had to act across each others rôles, a dependence on each other grew which made for a strong team. Small is beautiful did apply in the broadest sense, it was controllable and self sufficient.

In the main I felt the unit was well balanced on the

clinical, scientific and humanitarian fronts. Some volunteers dramatised their suffering at the hands of the virologist, but this did not get misquoted or taken out of context, or brought to the attention of the newspapes thus bringing the wrath of the public down on Harvard. The public relations carried out by the General Office and the Executive Officer over so many prevented and balanced any adverse criticism. By the time I joined Harvard the system was as streamlined and efficient as possible and paved the way for full co-operaton of the volunteers.

The impact Harvard had on me was the self discipline and dedication of the virologist, the life at Harvard as a volunteer or worker made for greater self sufficiency. I learnt how a few young people cannot cope well with their own company for ten days and if they could not stand their own company, then how could they expect others to put up with them!

The responsibility of being the only nurse on site was excellent experience in itself. Lastly some volunteers came to Harvard to escape stressful situations and were inclined to unburden their problems in talking to Matron. This made me develop an interest in counselling, which is important when caring for the disabled.

Miss Bailey is now the Matron of the Royal Star and Garter Home for Disabled Servicemen.

These experiences as a staff member relate not only to Miss Bailey but to other matrons both before and since she held the post.

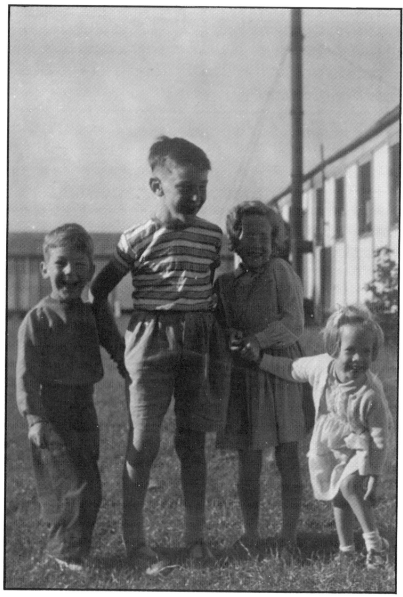

Children enjoying the open spaces at Harvard Hospital.

Appendix Three
The Harvard Children

The sign read "Drive Slowly beware of Children." It had been there almost from the first Trial. The child at the time was Ian Clarke, son of the Unit's chef. Ian was the first of approximately 40 children through the years to live at Harvard. Like the volunteers and staff they have always been accepted as part and parcel of the Harvard scene, much the same as children born and brought up on a farm or perhaps on a large private estate.

From taking their first steps to teenagers they respected the volunteer isolation procedures, never trespassing in that area confined to volunteers. Only when the volunteers had gone home did they venture into this "no go" playground which for ten days had been inviting to them.

I asked Frances and Susan Tyrrell who lived at Harvard in the 1950s — now married with children of their own — and ten year old Kerry and eight year old Alan Aldridge both born while dad was the Unit's Maintenance Engineer, and mum, a laboratory assistant, and who will be living at Harvard until the unit closes, for their memories and impressions.

First Frances and Susan:—

> When they first arrived families' meals were cooked in the central kitchen — they remember them being collected in large thermos containers, and they always seemed to be having suet pudding and custard for sweet. They both remember the dustbins being emptied each day by the porter with his electrically driven trolley rattling down the slatted walkways. Many hours were spent cycling along those same walkways that had odd sounding names. They crawled under the buildings and as a result were covered in chalk and cobwebs, finding dead hedgehogs and rabbits, some of which had carried

their offensive odour to the flat above. Playing in the old air raid shelters and Nissen huts, they found what seemed to them as children vast supplies left over from the War of unusual things such as Bibles, packs of poker playing cards, bars of soap, anti- gas capes, boxes of elastic bands, tongue depressors, blood transfusion kits, draughts and chess sets, American tin hats and old Christmas decorations to mention a few.

The girls mention their flat with windows of glass with wire netting embedded in them, the long corridor which they polished by dragging each other up and down on an old army blanket. Passing messages along on a piece of string from one bedroom to another attached to a ring.

Some members of the staff were more friendly to us than others. Miss Bullock the matron, Mickey the carpenter who gave us mugs of tea, Tom and Gladys who lived next door. On Sundays we sometimes fed the animals in the Unit's animal house with frozen meat. We gave the rabbits all names, "Bramble" was black, "Frosty" white, there was Big Ears, Loppy Ears, Junkie, Jim and Jean, remembering just a few.

The children often visited Mr Pike's farm next door with its cows, pigs, chicken and geese. Many would often stray into the Harvard grounds. They thought it fun rounding them up and returning them to the farm, not realising the damage they had sometimes caused.

During heavy downfalls of snow especially the 1962/63 winter when for two days no transport could negotiate the steep driveway they used metal trays as toboggans on the steeper slopes. It was great fun putting on Saturday shows in the small garage by their flat, dressing up to perform plays they had written themselves. Fetes were held with side-shows and selling cakes and coffee to raise money for charity.

The annual event they all looked forward to was Bonfire Night, for weeks beforehand everyone had helped the resident children to build the bonfire. A large crowd always came and the fireworks were lit with

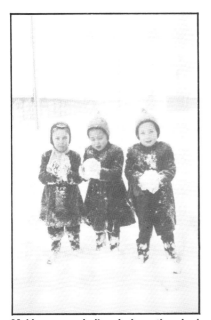

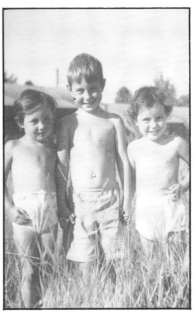

Making snowballs during the bad winter of 1962/63.

Children, stripped to the waist, during the summer.

safety in mind. It was their first experience of barbecued bacon, sausages and jacket potatoes.

They remember the embarrassment of not having a "proper" house to which they could bring their friends, but playing with them in their own vast private playground made up for it.

Each morning it was my job, using the unit's Mini Traveller to collect supplies for the kitchen. The children were taken to school at the same time. This quite often meant a tight squeeze. To ensure that the prime seats were not used by the same child each morning Frances drew a seating plan of the vehicle and a rota system was devised which caused much discussion among the children, all of which I found very amusing.

Kerry and Alan talk about similar experiences. Sadly they will be the last of the Harvard children, no others will enjoy the

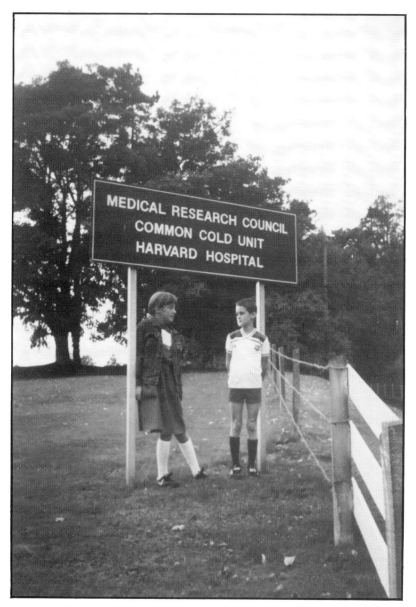

Kerry and Alan at the Common Cold Research Unit sign.

space and safety.

Kerry talks about the enjoyment of being able to "take off," sometimes to take a packed lunch and a blanket and to have a picnic out of site of their flat feeling they were picnicking miles from home. This they could not do anywhere else with the same feeling of safety and security.

All children enjoyed the availability of the many "Dens," summer dens, winter dens, wet weather dens, all to suit a child's imagination.

These, the last of the Harvard children still found odd bits and pieces of war-time leftovers, treasures to behold for growing and inquisitive children. Parents were not always pleased when their children returned home covered from head to toe in dirt and cobwebs, but soon became aware that visiting friends also enjoyed the unique experience of playing at Harvard and they soon wanted to return. When meeting the parents they often commented on how their off-springs talked non-stop about their day at Harvard, which often aroused my curiosity says Kerry and Alan's mum.

I don't remember any serious accident involving Harvard children, although there were one or two near misses. For example one lad climbed the ladder to the top of the water tower and was only seen when he panicked in trying to descend. The rescue was quite hazardous. On another occasion when children were having great fun pulling the garden roller to the top of a concrete slope and letting it free run down. A toddler, one of my own, strayed into its downward path and was snatched to safety at the last moment by his mother. As with children brought up on a farm with tractors there were a few tears from minor vehicle mishaps.

Christmas parties were held in the dining room, very often with a conjuror. Father Christmas visited the flats on Christmas morning. I think the adults enjoyed it just as much as the children.

Trips were organized to the local pantomime, piano lessons were given by Mrs Ray, the head cook's mother, Sunday School was held for a time in a nearby private house. When all was quiet and no other vehicles were using the roadways youngsters in their teens would be taught the rudiments of driving. Of course their was plenty of room for roller skating and in latter years skateboards. Children also enjoyed all manner of homemade "wheely" contraptions.

I'm sure eight year old Alan summed it all up for the Harvard children when he talked of looking across the fields surrounded by the many trees and if he sat quietly the rabbits would play around him and the birds would sit on the wires and he could watch the swallows nesting under the walkways. The thing he would miss most would be the space and again he mentioned the rabbits. When he was told that he would soon be moving he cried and said he didn't want to go and he would never forget Harvard.

These sentiments were also echoed by the daughters of Dr T. Sommerville who I met recently. Both were fond of riding and for a while had kept their horses at Harvard, when they moved to Scotland in 1951 they refused to speak to their parents and even threatened to run away back to Harvard.

Seal Island Supplies

SCHEDULE OF FOOD LOADED AT SALISBURY:—

Flour, white	420lb (6 sacks × 70lb)
Flour, wholemeal . .	410lb (6 sacks)
Biscuits, Army type . .	252lb (1 ctn × 28lb, 4 cases × 2 × 28lb)
Cream crackers . . .	15lb (3 tins × 5lb)
Savoury snacks . . .	8½lb (2 tines × 4¼lb)
Romany Parmistiks . .	7lb (2 tins × 3½lb)
Katherine biscuits . .	8¾lb (1 tin)
Fruit shortcake . . .	8lb (1 tin)
Lincoln cream . . .	7¼lb (1 tin)
Custard cream . . .	6¼lb (1 tin)
Vita Wheat	28lb (28 × 1lb pkts)
Suet, shredded . . .	12lb (12 × 1lb pkts)
Live poultry	24 head
	(together with 1 cwt of feeding stuff)
Corned beef	112lb (2 × 2lb, 3 cases 18 × 2lb)
Steak & kidney pudding	112lb (8 × 1lb, 2 cases 48 × 1lb)
Stewed steak	56lb (28 × 1lb, 20 × 1lb)
Ox tongue	12lb (2 × 6lb)
Boiled beef & carrots .	56lb (8 × 1lb, 1 case × 48 × 1lb)
Veal & ham	27lb (9 × 3lb)
Brisket of beef . . .	24lb (6 × 4lb)
Bacon, tinned	56lb (8 × 1lb, 1 case 48 × 1lb)
Sausage, tinned . . .	111lb (15 × 1lb, 2 cases × 48 × 1lb)
Potatoes, fresh . . .	336lb (3 sacks)
Potatoes, tinned . . .	248 tins (8 tins 20 ctns × 12 tins)
Potatoes, dehydrated .	60lb (3 cases × 2 × 10lb)
Eggs, preserved . . .	1080 No. (3 cases × 30 dozen)
Rice	7 lb (1 bag)
Macaroni	7lb (7 × 1lb)

Pearl barley	3lb (3 × 1lb)
Sago	4lb (4 × 1lb pkts)
Spaghetti	7lbg (7 × 1lb pkts)
Porridge pats	22lb (11 × 2lb pkts)
Cornflakes	21lb (28 × 12oz pkts)
Weetabix	14lb (287 × 8oz pkts)
Shredded wheat . . .	7lb (14 × 8oz pkts)
Puffed wheat	14lb (28 × 8oz pkts)
Butter, fresh	21lb (packets)
Butter, tinned . . .	35lb (35 × 1lb tins)
Margarine, fresh . . .	28lb (packets)
Margarine, tinned . .	28lb (28 × 1lb tins)
Lard	20lb (1 ctn × 4 × 5lb)
Frying oil	7lb (1 case × 7lb)
Cheese, English . . .	29lb (1 piece)
Processed Gruyere . .	10lb (20 boxes × 8oz)
Milk, condensed unsweetened	
F.C. 16oz tins . . .	624 tins (26 ctns × 24 tins)
Milk, condensed sweetened	
Skimmed	48 tins (1 ctn)
Jam, plum	24lb (1 ctn × 12 × 2lb)
Jam, apricot	24lb (1 ctn × 12 × 2lb)
Jam, strawberry . . .	24lb (1 ctn × 12 × 2lb)
Marmalade	28lb (4 × 2lb 10 × 2lb)
Golden syrup	28lb (14 × 2lb)
Lemon curd	14lb (14 × 1lb)
Sugar, granulated . .	91lb (1 sack × 50lb 1 sack × 41lb)
Sugar, Demarara . .	14lb (1 bag)
Sugar, caster	7lb (7 × 1lb)
Sugar, icing	7lb (7 × 1lb)
Apples	
Oranges	
Dates	7lb
Raisins	3lb (1 case)
Sultanas	4lb
Figs	7lb
Prunes	14lb (1 case)
Currants	7lb

Apple rings   .   .   .   .   14lb (1 case)
Cherries, tinned .   .   .   8lb (4 × 2lb)
Pears, tinned .   .   .   .   24lb (12 × 2lb)
Peaches, tinned .   .   .   12lb (6 × 2lb)
Plums, tinned   .   .   .
Plums, bottled   .   .   .
Egg, dried .   .   .   .   .   8¾lb (28 × 5oz tins)
Carrots, fresh 112lb
Carrots, tinned   .   .   .   28lb (6 tins 1 ctn × 12 tins)
Beetroot, tinned .   .   .   50lb (1 tin 1 case × 24 tins)
Peas, tinned .   .   .   .   60lb (6 tins 1 case × 24 tins)
Celery, tinned   .   .   .   28lb (1 case × 18 tins)
Parsnips, tinned .   .   .   30lb (4 tins 1 case × 12 tins)
Macedoine, tinned .   .   10lb (6 tins)
Beans in tomato sauce .   28lb (4 tins 1 ctn × tins)
Tomatoes, tinned   .   .   30lb (1 case × 15 tins)
Beans, Haricot   .   .   .   10lb (1 bag)
Peas, marrowfat .   .   .   14lb (1 bag)
Lentils .   .   .   .   .   .   4lb (1 ctn)
Onions 168lb
Herrings, tinned .   .   .   28lb (28 × 1lb)
Salmon, tinned   .   .   .   15lb (15 × 1lb (grade II))
Sardines, tinned .   .   .   7lb (28 × 4oz tins)
Crawfish .   .   .   .   .   4lb (16 × 4oz tins)
Tea .   .   .   .   28lb (3lb 1 case × 25lb)
Cocoa, Bournville   .   .   6lb (6 × 1lb tins)
Cocoa, fortified   .   .   .   4lb (2 × 2lb)
    (Ostermilk tins with tape on)
Salt, cooking .   .   .   .   14lb (1 bag)
Salt, table .   .   .   .   .   14lb (15 tins)
Mustard, powdered   .   ½lb
Mustard, French .   .   .   ½lb (4 × 2oz jars)
Vinegar   .   .   .   .   .   1 gal (1 jar in wicker basket)
Baking powder   .   .   .   6lb (2 ctns × 12 × 4oz tins)
Custard powder .   .   .   3lb (4 × 12oz tins)
Cornflour .   .   .   .   .   3lb (3 × 1lb bags)
Blancmange powder   .   2lb (24 pkts)
Pickles

Chef brown onion	.	4 × 10oz jars
Chef mixed pickles	.	4 × 10 oz jars
Chef green label chutney	.	12 × 10oz jars
C. & B. Picalilli . .	.	2 × 10oz jars
Heinz Ideal Pickle	.	2 × 10oz jars

Sauces

H.P.	.	9 bottles
Tomato ketchup .	.	9 bottles
Worcester . . .	.	3 bottles
Anchovery essence .		3 bottles
Coffee, ground . .	.	15lb (5 × 3lb)
Nescafé	.	4lb (4 × 1lb tins)
Yeast, dried . .	.	15lb (15 × 1lb tins)
Tablets, Multivite .	.	2000 No. (2 bottles × 1000)
Fish paste	.	48 jars
Meat paste . . .	.	24 jars
Sandwich spread	.	24 jars (1 ctn)
Salad cream . . .	.	24 jars (1 ctn)
Essence, almond . .	.	1 bottle
Essence, vanilla . .	.	1 bottle
Essence, lemon . .	.	1 bottle
Saccharine		3000 No. (3 bottles × 1000 tablets)
Curry powder . .	.	3lb
Nutmegs, whole . .	.	6
Cinnamon	.	¼lb (4 × 1oz drums)
Mixed spice . . .	.	½lb
Ginger, ground . .	.	½lb
Paxo stuffing . . .	.	18 pkts
Soups, tinned . .	.	48 tins (1 case)
Soups, powdered asstd .		10lb (10 × 1lb)
Bovril	.	2lb (2 × 16oz jars)
Marmite	.	2lb (2 × 16oz jars)
Mixed peel . . .	.	1lb
Gravy browning . .	.	1 bottle
Cream of tartar . .	.	1lb
Soya flour	.	2lb
Jelly tablets		72 × 1 pt size

Lemonade crystals,
  Eiffel Tower . . . 6 tins
Lemon barley crystals .   12 tins
Treacle puddings, tinned 48 tins (1 ctn)
Walnuts . . . . . 28lb (1 bag)

Invalid diet:—
  Ovaltine . . . 3 tins
  Powdered Milk . . 3 tins (Ostermilk)
  Glucose . . . . . 2 tins

Packing Inventory

Bin No. 3	6 buckets G.I., 1 scales, kitchen 1 knife, carving 1 fork, flesh, 2 saws, bread, 1 pin, rolling, 2 knives, slicing, 1 spatula, 1 ladle, soup, 1 whisk 12in 2 spoons, wooden 16in.
1 Bin No. 1	2 extincteurs S/A empty, 2 extincteurs C.T.C. filled, 2 charges, spare C.T.C., 6 hanging brackets for Aladdin lamps, 6 hooks for Aladdin lamps, 6 reflectors for Aladdin lamps, 4 brushes, nail, 3 brushes, bannister, soft, 3 pkts towels, paper, 6 bars soap, scouring.
1 carton "Hygiene Stores"	1 tin Ratbane, 1 tin varnish (rat & mouse), 6 pieces cardboard, 6 mousetraps, 1 rat trap, 1 sprayer "Monitor", 3 tins powder D.D.T., 1lb Permanganate of potash, 6 tins Izal powder, 10 balls twine, 5 balls cord, 3 yds butter muslin.
1 × 5 gal drum	D.D.T. solution
1 × 2 gal can	Dettol
1 × 2 gal drum	Disinfectant
1	Stretcher & Thomas splint
1 pannier	Field Medical No. 1

1 pannier	Field Medical No. 2
1 carton marked	"Medical" containing 3 haversacks surgical, 1 set testing water, sterilization.
1 incinerator	6 bukets fire, 1 kettle aluminium, 3 racks, cake, 2 boards, bread.
2 valises	7 camp beds complete, 7 bags for beds, 3 wash-stands, 3 bags for wash-stands, 3 wash-basins, 1 bucket, canvas, 3 ground sheets.
4 tables	Folding 4ft 6in
2 table	Canteen 7ft
4 cupboards	Folded flat
8 chairs	Canvas arm
3 bundles	10 deck chairs
1 oven marked "1"	Shelf, rack, deflector plate, lifter, instruction card, 1 tin baking, 3 dishes pie E.I., 2 tins Swiss roll, 2 tins pâté, 4 tins flan, 4 tins sandwich, 1 roaster with lid, 2 slices fish, 2 spoons gravy.
1 oven marked "2"	Shelf, rack, deflector plate, lifter, instruction card, 1 tin baking, 1 roaster with lid, 2 tin-openers, 2 corkscrews, 1 knife sharpener, 2 potato peeler/apple corers, 1 brush pastry, 1 grater, 8 tins, bread 2lb, 1 set pastry cutters.
1 carton "Night"	4 pots chamber, 1 brush wall 5in, 2 × 1pt white paint.
Carton "Primus"	4 stoves Coleman "Solus" (2 fitted with No. 5 burners, 2 fitted with No. 10 burners), 2 burners spare No. 10, 2 burners spare No. 5, 2 nipples No. 5, 1 key nipple No. 5, 6 pkts needles cleaning No. 5, 2 washers, pump 2 washers, filler cap, 4 nipples No. 10, 1 key nipple No. 10, 7 pkts needles cleaning No. 10, 6 washers, burner 3 funnels 2 draught excluders.

Bin No. 2	2 bowls mixing E.I., 1 colander, 1 pot boiling aluminium, 3 tins cake, 1 sieve flour, 1 bin, scrap with lid, 1 pkt towels paper, 1 bowl E.I., 2 scourers pot, 3lb soap yellow, 1 sieve, gravy, 1 measure, graduated aluminium.
1 carton marked 1st Week "B"	Assorted foodstuffs.
1 sack	Wholemeal flour.
2 cartons	Evaporated milk
1 carton marked 1st Week "A"	Assorted foodstuffs.
1 carton	Tea and marmalade
1 carton	Golden plums
1 sack	Sugar
1 case	30 dozen eggs
1 carton	Apricot jam
1 carton	Tinned meats
1 case	Sausage
1 case	Dried fruit
1 bag	Marrowfat peas
1 carton	Lard
1 plywood box containing 5 cartons marked "GLASS"	9 plates dinner, 9 plates soup, 9 plates tart, 9 plates tea, 4 plates bread and butter, 9 saucers, 9 cups tea, 3 cups egg, 9 glasses ½pt, 4 teapots 2½pt E/W, 2 basins sugar, 4 jugs 1pt e/w, 4 jugs 2pt e/w, 1 jug 4pt E/W, 18 spoons soup, 18 spoons tea, 4 spoons table, 18 forks dessert, 18 knives dessert, 3 sets condiment, 3 strainers tea, 2 × 1000 Multivite tablets, 1 box applicators wood, 4 charges S/A, 2 lamps Bialaddin complete, 6 glasses for Aladdin lamps.
Bin No. 4	6 founts Aladdin, 6 burners Aladdin, 12 mantles Aladdin, 2yds wick,

	Hurricane lamp, 2 lamps, electric cycle, 12 batteries spare, 9 cloths sponge, 5 cloths floor, 2 pkts towels paper.
Bin No. 6	2 saucepans, E/I 6pt, 1 saucepan aluminium with lid, 2 kettles E/I 5pt, 1 bowl E/I, 3 toasters (for primus).
Bin No. 7	1 tripod, primus, 3 trays, 1 poacher egg 7 hole, 14lb powder scouring, 1 last cobbling, 1 set shoe repair gear.
1 wicker basket	2 bins bread, 1 saucepan E/I 10in, 1 pan frying large, 1 pan frying 10in, 1 steel butchers, 1 knife sharpener carborundum, 1 container square E/I with lid, 1 container tin 14lb, 3 containers tin (ex-thermos jars), 3 basins E/W 4pt, 1 bath oval E/I, 2 dishes meat E/I, 1 roll paper greaseproof, 5lb soap yellow, 10 doz (approx) outfits insect repellant, 4 sheets cot (for tablecloths), 7 cloths glass, 2 slips pillow, 4 towel face, 2 yds waterproof sheeting, 1 kettle iron 12pt.
1 carton marked "Steamer"	1 steamer 2 tier with lid, 2 saucepans E/I 6pt, 1 glass for lamp Bialaddin, 6 mantles for lamp Bialaddin, 1 set washer for lamp Bialaddin, 1 vaporiser for lamp Bialaddin, 1 purer methylated spirits, 20 yds heavy rope, 40 yds calf rope, 1 axe hand, 1 tin Dubbin.
Bath No. 1	1 coco square (bath mat), 8 mats (bedside), 1 wringer, 2 bath tidies, 12 boxes soap, 6 bowls E/I, 1 baler handled, 5 pkts towels paper, 1 tin Calgon (water softener), 1 saw hand, 5 golf clubs, 1 cricket bat, 1 set stumps, 1 fishing rod (Mr Betteridge).
Bath No. 2	5 mats (bedside), 1 coco square (bath

mat), 2 baths oval E/I, 2 buckets E/I, 1 tin Calgon (water softener), 1 holder paper towels, 1 pkt towels paper, 12 ashtrays, 2 jugs E/I 2pt, 2 jugs E/I 4pt, 1 saw Bushmans, 1 spade, 1 fork, 1 hoe, 1 rake, 1 trowel, 1 fork hand, 7lb lime, 7lb Nationa Growmore, 1pt mustard seed, 1pt cress, 1oz raddish seed, ½oz lettuce seed.

Lifebuoy and 5lb coil wire galvanised.

1 meat safe	
1 boiler 10 gal	7lb wool waste, 5lb rags cleaning.
1 washing machine	2 flat irons, 1 ironing blanket, 1 clothes line, 72 pegs, 1 iron cover, 12lb soap yellow, 24 pkts powder detergent, 3 laundry blue.
1 carton marked "Stationery"	Assorted stationery and C.C.R.U. forms, haircutting outfit.
1 case marked "Library"	Books
1 carton "Welfare"	Assorted games & handicraft materials
42 cases	Foodstuffs (see consignment note)
76 cartons	Foodstuffs (see consignment note)
16 sacks	Foodstuffs (see consignment note)
4 bags	Foodstuffs (see consignment note)
3 Pkgs of tins	Foodstuffs (see consignment note)
1 container insulated	Foodstuffs (see consignment note)
1 wicker basket	Foodstuffs (see consignment note)
2 sheets plywood	For use as table tennis table.

Note: E/W = Earthenware. E/I = Enamelled Iron.

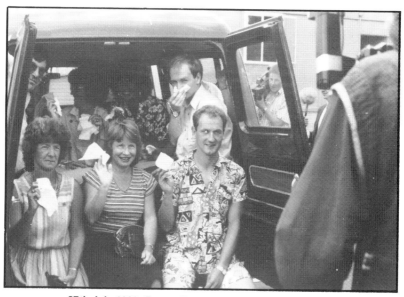

27th July 1989: Farewell to the last Harvard volunteers.

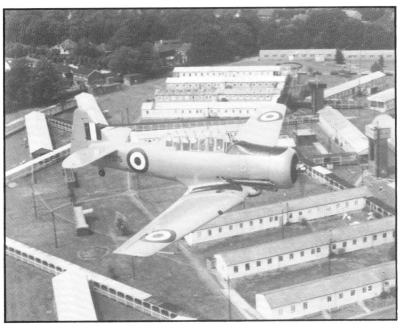

Harvard Trainer dipping wings in salute on the closure of its namesake (Crown Copyright/A&AEE Photograph, reproduced by permission of the Controller of Her Majesty's Stationery Office).

Paean To Harvard

Last night you, a unit, died, life all gone,
A lonely doctor walked through empty corridors.
Echoes of past laughter ringing in his ears.

Infancy brought from a far land,
No price too high was an ocean graveyard.
The trees that grew so long ago reaching to
Heaven in that continent across the sea
Lived on in hutted complexity,
Keeping their secrets of brave men, long forgotten —
Physicians, nurses, and whom

Your adolescence came, to
This part of Salisbury Plain,
When battle commenced against the cold war
From an Idealist now resting in our halls of fame.

You blossomed and grew and became famous too
With soldiers of science, helpers, volunteers,
Over forty three years.
Great discoveries made — international repute
Could not save you from the ultimate shoot.
New young life may spring from your acres
Mingling their laughter with ghosts of the past

Spirit of Harvard sail on in the wind
Hold your head high
You were the greatest — though you had to die.

Written by Matron Mrs Ann Dalton

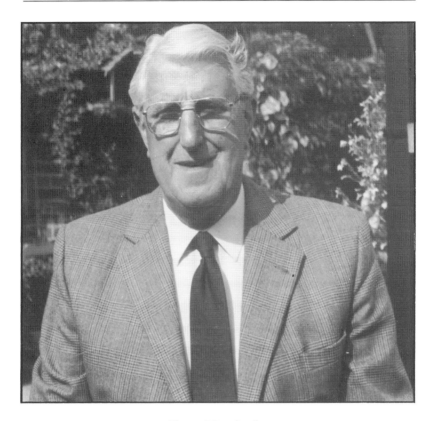

About The Author

Keith Thompson was born in Norfolk. Following his demobilisation from the Services in April 1946 he commenced work as a driver to the Medical Council in London, but soon transferred to Harvard Hospital, on the outskirts of Salisbury. From 1946 to 1982 he was employed at Harvard and was ultimately involved with administration work at the hospital. He was present when the first group of volunteers arrived on 17th July 1946 and was, again, present when the last group of volunteers left on 27th July 1989. Keith Thompson now lives in retirement at Salisbury, not far from the site of Harvard Hospital. He is married with two sons, and lists furniture-making among his hobbies.